T0180189

Coronary Vasomotion Abnormalities

Hiroaki Shimokawa

Editor

Coronary Vasomotion Abnormalities

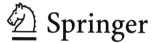 Springer

Editor
Hiroaki Shimokawa
Department of Cardiovascular Medicine
Tohoku University Graduate School of Medicine
Sendai
Miyagi
Japan

ISBN 978-981-15-7596-9   ISBN 978-981-15-7594-5   (eBook)
https://doi.org/10.1007/978-981-15-7594-5

This Springer imprint is published by the registered company Springer Nature Singapore Pte Ltd.
The registered company address is: 152 Beach Road, #21-01/04 Gateway East, Singapore 189721, Singapore

Preface

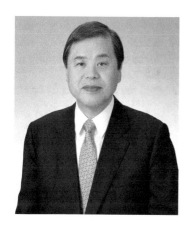

Stable coronary artery disease (CAD) is mainly caused by the various combinations of the three mechanisms, including epicardial organic coronary stenosis, epicardial coronary artery spasm, and coronary microvascular dysfunction (CMD). The representative manifestations of those three mechanisms are effort angina, vasospastic angina (VSA), and microvascular angina (MVA), respectively. Among them, VSA and MVA represent typical manifestations of coronary functional abnormalities. To date, much attention has been paid to the first mechanism, epicardial organic coronary stenosis, leading to the successful developments of percutaneous coronary intervention (PCI) and coronary artery bypass grafting (CABG). However, it is also widely known that approximately 40% of patients with obstructive CAD still suffer from persistent/recurrent angina even after complete revascularization with PCI and/or CABG. Also, the prevalence of angina with non-obstructive CAD has been rapidly increasing worldwide, approximately 70% in women and 50% in men. Furthermore, to the surprise of the world, recently, the ISCHEMIA Trial has convincingly demonstrated that revascularization strategy with PCI or CABG has no prognostic benefit in patients with stable CAD with proven moderate to severe myocardial ischemia (*NEJM*, 2020). These lines of evidence indicate the importance of coronary artery vasomotion abnormalities in the pathogenesis of stable CAD.

In 1983, I succeeded in developing the first animal model of coronary artery spasm in pigs (*Science*, 1983) and have been performing a series of experimental and clinical studies since then for almost 40 years. My research group has demonstrated that coronary spasm is caused mainly by vascular smooth muscle hypercontraction mediated by Rho-kinase activation, that chronic adventitial inflammation is a central pathophysiology of the spasm, and that Rho-kinase inhibitor, fasudil, is very effective for the spasm. We have also performed domestic and international collaboration registry studies on coronary artery spasm, demonstrating the ethnic differences in clinical characteristics, treatments, and long-term prognosis of VSA patients.

We have also performed a series of experimental and clinical studies on CMD, in which we demonstrated that Rho-kinase activation also plays an important role in the pathogenesis of CMD and that epicardial spasm and CMD frequently co-exist. As a member of the Coronary Vasomotion Disorders International Study Group (COVADIS), I have also been performing an international prospective registry study on MVA, which demonstrated the ethnic differences in clinical patient characteristics, treatments, and long-term prognosis of MVA patients.

After almost 40 years of research, I have retired from Tohoku University in March 2020 and planned to publish a book that summarizes research works mainly from my laboratory to memorize my research on coronary vasomotion abnormalities. In Part I, we will focus on epicardial coronary artery spasm, including epidemiology of VSA, and pathophysiology, molecular mechanisms, diagnosis, and treatment of coronary artery spasm. In Part II, we will focus on CMD, including its epidemiology, pathophysiology, diagnosis, and treatment.

I hope that this book will help readers better understand the progress and current knowledge on coronary vasomotion abnormalities.

Sendai, Miyagi, Japan   Hiroaki Shimokawa

Contents

Part I
Epicardial Coronary Artery Spasm

Chapter 1
Epidemiology of Vasospastic Angina

Jun Takahashi and Hiroaki Shimokawa

Abstract Vasospastic angina (VSA) is one of the important functional cardiac disorders characterized by transient myocardial ischemia due to epicardial coronary artery spasm. The term of VSA is basically synonymous with the terms Prinzmetal's angina and variant angina, and is known to be associated with a wide variety of cardiac ischemic conditions, including stable angina, acute coronary syndrome, and life-threatening arrhythmic events. A number of studies have elucidated patient characteristics, outcomes, and prognostic factors of VSA, which led to a better understanding and management for this disorder. However, there remains to be insufficient data on the prevalence of VSA in both Eastern and Western countries, probably because it is difficult and cumbersome to examine coronary spasm during coronary angiography. On the other hand, it has been well known that age, smoking, high-sensitivity C-reactive protein, and remnant lipoprotein are significant risk factors for coronary spasm. Recently, the Japanese Coronary Spasm Association (JCSA) demonstrated that, in the temporary VSA patients, overall 5-year survival rate free from all-cause death or major adverse cardiac events was 98% and 91%, indicating the clinical outcome appears to be further improved as compared with the 1980s. Furthermore, the JCSA also developed a risk scoring system consisting of 7 predictive factors including history of out-of-hospital cardiac arrest and smoking, of which the average prediction rate was approximately 90%. In this chapter, we will briefly review the epidemiological data regarding VSA from a broad set of perspectives, including demographic characteristics, incidence and prognosis, risk and precipitating factors, and other recent clinical topics.

Keywords Prevalence · Prognosis · Risk factors · Predictive factors · Sudden cardiac death · Racial difference

J. Takahashi · H. Shimokawa (✉)
Department of Cardiovascular Medicine, Tohoku University Graduate School of Medicine, Sendai, Miyagi, Japan
e-mail: shimo@cardio.med.tohoku.ac.jp

1.1   Coronary Artery Spasm and Coronary Ischemic Syndromes

Angina pectoris is a clinical syndrome caused by transient myocardial ischemia due to an imbalance between myocardial oxygen demand and supply [1]. For more than 200 years since the description by Heberdenk, its pathogenesis has been explained by increased myocardial oxygen demand in the presence of fixed organic stenosis of the epicardial coronary arteries. Angina caused by spasm of epicardial coronary arteries has been known as variant angina. By most strict definition, variant angina is a diagnosis given to patients having rest angina associated with reversible ST-segment elevation on electrocardiogram (ECG) but no evidence of myocardial necrosis as determined by serial ECGs and enzymatic analysis. This peculiar form of angina pectoris was systematically described for the first time by Myron Prinzmetal and colleagues in 1959, based on the observations of 32 patients with rest angina associated with transient ST elevation [2]. All characteristic clinical features that are at present well recognized were mostly reported in the Prinzmetal report. Namely, chest pain typically occurs at midnight or in the early hours of the morning and tends to be clustered. Night awakening with chest pain is also common. As compared with classical angina, chest pain in variant angina is usually longer in duration and severe in intensity, and frequently associated with autonomic symptoms such as nausea and cold sweating. In general, the patients do not develop angina on exertion unless obstructive coronary atherosclerosis is concomitantly present and exercise tolerance during daytime is usually preserved. Shortly after the Prinzmetal report, coronary artery spasm was angiographically documented by Gensini et al. in a patient with rest and effort angina [3]. Furthermore, in the 1970s, Yasue et al. demonstrated spasm of an epicardial coronary artery during an attack of variant angina systematically induced by methacholine or exercise in the early morning [4, 5]. Endo et al. also reported similar findings almost simultaneously [6]. Coronary angiography during anginal attacks in patients suffering from recurrent angina at rest revealed a wide range of coronary artery disease from normal coronaries to severe three-vessel disease. ST-segment elevation was caused by a transient occlusion of the major coronary artery, whereas ST depression was caused by incomplete occlusion of coronary branches and invariably associated with the extensive coronary artery disease and rich collateral networks. Coronary collaterals develop with or without coronary artery disease and can modify the extent and severity of myocardial ischemia [7, 8]. Spasm of large epicardial coronary arteries causes angina at rest associated with ST elevation [3] or depression [7, 9]. Then, variant angina is now regarded as one aspect of the wide spectrum of myocardial ischemic syndromes caused by coronary spasm, and angina pectoris caused by coronary spasm is generally called vasospastic angina (VSA).

In addition to rest angina, coronary artery spasm plays a pivotal role in a broad spectrum of coronary ischemic syndrome, including exercise-induced angina, silent myocardial ischemia, pre-infarction (unstable) angina, acute myocardial infarction, postinfarction angina, syncope, and sudden cardiac death (Fig. 1.1) [10]. Especially,

Fig. 1.1 Coronary artery spasm has been shown to play a key role in the pathogenesis of not only variant angina but also a number of related conditions in ischemic heart disease. (Reproduced from Takagi et al. [36])

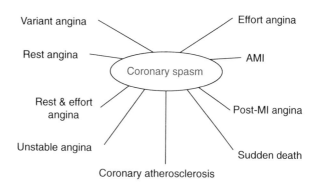

coronary artery spasm can also be the cause of effort angina. It was generally believed that exercise-induced angina was caused by increased myocardial oxygen demand in the presence of flow-limiting organic stenosis and that ST elevation during exercise testing indicated the presence of severe organic stenosis. Coronary angiograms taken during exercise in the cardiac catheterization laboratory clearly demonstrated that exercise provoked coronary artery spasm, leading to total obstruction of major coronary artery at the site of no significant organic stenosis at baseline [11, 12]. The elevation or depression of ST-segment during exercise may be determined by the severity and extent of coronary artery spasm, the underlying coronary artery disease, or both [7, 13, 14].

It should be noted that patients with VSA often exhibit a marked variability of exercise capacity even in the same day. The circadian variation in angina threshold is an important diagnostic clue to suspect the involvement of coronary spasm in ischemic manifestations. It was shown that epicardial coronary artery tone as well as the sensitivity of coronary arteries to vasoconstrictor stimuli (e.g. ergonovine) varied substantially in the morning and in the afternoon [11, 15]. The underlying mechanism of the circadian variation is not fully understood, but may be related, at least partly, to the changes in the activity of autonomic nervous system [16, 17], endothelial function [18], and Rho-kinase activity [19]. The results based on the 24-h ambulatory ECG monitoring have shown that silent myocardial ischemia is frequently observed in patients with variant angina and approximately 80% of ischemia with transient ST elevation was asymptomatic [20]. Silent ischemia was associated with malignant ventricular tachyarrhythmias and may cause sudden cardiac death [21, 22].

In a subset of patients, coronary artery spasm is responsible for acute coronary thrombosis, resulting in pre-infarction unstable angina and acute myocardial infarction. It was previously reported that intracoronary nitroglycerin was effective to recanalize occluded vessel by relieving spasm in 6 out of 15 patients with acute myocardial infarction within 12 h after the onset [23]. In all the 6 patients, spasm was superimposed on the high-grade atherosclerotic stenosis. This result suggests that coronary spasm might be the primary cause of acute coronary occlusion or, at least, the secondary event to sustain flow impairment. Not rarely, myocardial infarction develops in the absence of significant organic stenosis [24, 25]. It was also shown that coronary spasm could be provoked at 4 weeks after the onset in 75% of patients with acute myocardial infarction (AMI) and no significant organic stenosis in Japan [25]. These patients were characterized by the presence of pre-infarction and/or postin-farction angina at rest, the occurrence of multivessel spasm, and smaller infarct size. According to a recent study from Germany, in which the frequency of coronary spasm in patients with acute coronary syndrome (ACS) and unobstructed coronary arteries was examined by the intracoronary acetylcholine provocation test, every forth patients with ACS had no culprit lesion and almost 50% of the patients who underwent a provocation testing had proof of coronary spasm [26]. In general, postin-farction angina is a predictor of adverse outcomes after AMI [27]. However, coronary spasm is the cause of postinfarction angina in a subset of patients with cyclic ST elevation and they may have no critical stenosis on angiography [28, 29]. In almost of them, calcium channel blockers (e.g. diltiazem) are effective and the prognosis is generally favorable. Provocation testing frequently provokes coronary spasms in patients with AMI. When the relationship between provoked coronary spasm and clinical course in AMI patients was examined, the frequency of major adverse car-diac event-free survival was significantly higher in the positive group than in the negative group [30]. These results indicate that provoked coronary spasm is a signifi-cant independent predictor of poor prognosis in AMI patients.

1.2 Prevalence of Vasospastic Angina

There are insufficient data on the prevalence of VSA in both Eastern and Western countries, probably because it is difficult and cumbersome to examine coronary spasm during coronary angiography. To determine the prevalence of VSA, a survey was conducted on 2251 consecutive patients with angina (average age of 65.2 years) hospitalized in 15 major cardiovascular medical institutions in Japan in 1998 [31]. The survey showed that about 40% of patients with angina in Japan had VSA. Furthermore, analysis of the age group distribution of VSA revealed that the prevalence tended to be higher in relatively young patients than in elderly one. Recently, however, increase in use rate of calcium channel blockers (CCBs) for hypertension as well as decreasing rates of smoking might result in decreased mor-bidity of VSA in Japan [32]. It has been long believed that the prevalence of VSA patients is higher in Japanese than in Caucasian populations [33, 34]. This concept is consistent with a head-to-head controlled comparison of patients with acute ST elevation AMI (without a history of VSA) where Japanese patients were twice as likely to have inducible spasm than their Caucasian counterparts [35]. Furthermore, in Western studies, the diagnosis of VSA is primarily made on the basis of spontane-ous episodes (i.e. anginal symptoms with ischemic ECG changes), whereas in Japan, it is more often based upon spasm provocation testing [36]. However, it has been recently demonstrated that the prevalence of coronary artery spasm in Caucasians may be higher than previously thought [37, 38]. Indeed, while previous Asian studies of patients without obstructive coronary artery disease have shown that the prevalence of coronary spasm was ~50% in patients with stable angina and

57% in patients with acute coronary syndrome [39, 40]; similar findings were demonstrated in Germany studies [26, 37]. Furthermore, Ong et al. demonstrated that, among 921 consecutive white patients with angina and nonobstructive coronary arteries, the overall frequency of epicardial spasm was 33.4%, and that of microvascular spasm was 24.2%, indicating that the morbidity of coronary functional disorder including VSA may be higher than we thought [41].

1.3 Risk Factors and Precipitating Factors for Coronary Artery Spasm

Age, smoking, high-sensitivity C-reactive protein (hsCRP), and remnant lipoprotein are significant risk factors for coronary spasm [42–45]. Generally, VSA is a disease of middle- and elderly aged men and postmenopausal women [42, 46]. Meanwhile, cigarette smoking, which has been identified as a risk factor for coronary artery spasm in various groups of patients including premenopausal women [47–49], has a strong effect on VSA development in younger than in their old counterparts [50, 51]. Nicotine potently upregulates Rho-kinase, which has been identified as one of the effectors of the small GTP-binding protein Rho and plays a key role in the molecular mechanisms of VSA, in human coronary artery smooth muscle cells, while estrogens potently downregulate it [52, 53]. Smoking is a controllable factor in preventing the development of coronary spasm and cessation of smoking is associated with spontaneous remission of angina [54]. High LDL cholesterol and insulin resistance were suggested to be a risk factor for VSA in selected patients [48, 55], but were not confirmed by others. Furthermore, it also has been suggested that oxidative stress may be associated with abnormalities of triglyceride metabolism and HDL cholesterol level reduction [20, 56]. However, the role of dyslipidemia as a risk factor for coronary spasm remains to be less clear. Thus, except for smoking, many conventional risk factors for atherosclerosis appear to be insignificant for VSA. On the other hand, it was reported that serum levels of hsCRP were elevated in VSA patients than in non-VSA patients [57] and that 6-month treatment with a statin could significantly reduce the disease activity of VSA along with the decrease in hsCRP levels [58]. These results suggest that low-grade inflammation caused by risk factors including smoking and hyperlipidemia is involved in the pathogenesis of VSA and that hsCRP is useful for disease activity assessment of VSA.

1.4 Prognosis and Predictive Factors for Vasospastic Angina

The prevalence of major adverse cardiac events (MACE) in VSA is difficult to define because of the variation in defining the disorder. Several important prognostic studies with a few hundreds of patients were performed in the 1980s. Shimokawa et al. reported that overall survival rates at 1, 3, and 5 years among consecutive 158

Japanese patients with variant angina were 99, 96, and 93%, respectively, and survival rates without AMI at 1, 3, and 5 years were 94, 92, and 87%, respectively [59]. Yasue et al. also reported that 5-year survival rate free from death or myocardial infarction was 97% and 83% in 245 patients [60]. On the other hand, the prognosis of Caucasian population of the day was much worse, demonstrating that 5-year survival rate free from death or myocardial infarction was 89% and 69%, respectively [61]. In association with the epidemics of obesity and metabolic syndrome, the general population has been rapidly growing older and the Westernization of lifestyle has been progressing, especially in Japan [62]. Thus, we conducted the nationwide multicenter retrospective registry study by the Japanese Coronary Spasm Association (JCSA), which focused on the clinical characteristics and outcomes of VSA patients in the 2000s (Fig. 1.2) [36]. During the median follow-up period of 32 months, among 1429 patients with VSA, 19 (1.3%) died, in which 6 had cardiac death. MACE occurred in 85 patients (5.9%), including AMI ($n = 9$), hospitalization for unstable angina ($n = 68$) and heart failure ($n = 4$), and appropriate ICD shocks ($n = 2$). Overall 5-year survival rate free from all cause death or MACE was 98% and 91%, respectively (Fig. 1.3) [36]. Especially, 5-year survival rate free from nonfatal AMI was high (99%). Moreover, Ong et al. reported that ACS patients without culprit lesion and proven coronary spasm have an excellent prognosis for survival and coronary events after 3 years compared with those with obstructive

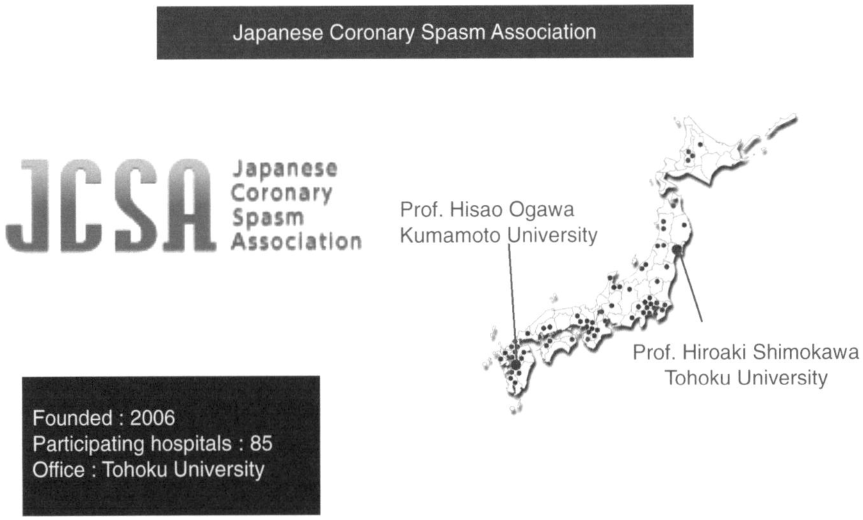

Fig. 1.2 The Japanese Coronary Spasm Association (JCSA) was established in 2006 by Prof. Shimokawa and Ogawa to elucidate the clinical characteristics and outcomes of patients with VSA in the current era and conducted the nationwide multicenter registry study of VSA

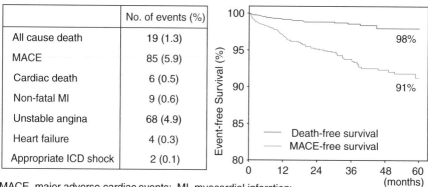

	No. of events (%)
All cause death	19 (1.3)
MACE	85 (5.9)
Cardiac death	6 (0.5)
Non-fatal MI	9 (0.6)
Unstable angina	68 (4.9)
Heart failure	4 (0.3)
Appropriate ICD shock	2 (0.1)

MACE, major adverse cardiac events; MI, myocardial infarction;
ICD, implantable cardioverter defibrillator.

Fig. 1.3 Clinical outcomes of 1429 VSA patients enrolled into the nationwide multicenter retrospective registry study by the Japanese Coronary Spasm Association. During the median follow-up period of 32 months, 19 patients (1.3%) died and MACE occurred in 85 patients. Overall 5-year survival rate free from all cause death or MACE was 98% and 91%, respectively. (Reproduced from Takagi et al. [36])

ACS [63]. Taken together, in the current era, the clinical outcome of VSA patients appears to be further improved as compared with the 1980s. It is important to continue medical treatments with CCB for VSA, since silent myocardial ischemia with fatal arrhythmia and a rebound phenomenon of the spasm could occur after withdrawal of CCB [21, 64].

Several prognostic factors for VSA, such as smoking, organic coronary stenosis, and multivessel spasm, have been established since the 1980s [59–61, 65–67]. Recently, in addition to the aforementioned prognostic factors, we newly identified the prognostic impact of history of out-of-hospital cardiac arrest (OHCA) [36] and specific angiographic findings during the diagnostic provocation tests [68]. However, in order to apply such prognostic findings to clinical practice, the accumulation of various prognostic factors in individual patients should be taken into consideration. Additionally, it is conceivable that potential interactions among those prognostic factors exist, making it difficult to assess individual prognosis. Thus, we developed the JCSA risk scoring system as a comprehensive assessment tool that provides the valid risk prediction in individual patients [69]. This JCSA risk score, which consists of 7 predictive factors, including history of OHCA, smoking, angina at rest alone, significant organic stenosis, multivessel spasm, ST-segment elevation during angina, and β-blocker use, showed a significant correlation with the prognosis of VSA patients (see Chap. 4, Fig. 4.3a, b). The average prediction rate of the scoring system was approximately 90%, suggesting that the risk scoring system could accurately estimate future adverse cardiac events in individual VSA patient. Since the clinical information required for the scoring system is readily available from routine practice, it should help clinicians predict patient outcomes easily. The information on the prognostic stratification may lead to personalized management, including the judgment of necessity for intensive medical treatment and close follow-up. In addition, because the outcomes of VSA patients could be aggravated by a rebound phenomenon after careless discontinuation of medications [36, 64], it is of clinical significance that the adherence in high-risk patients should be improved through the awareness with this risk score.

1.5   Sudden Cardiac Death in Vasospastic Angina

Syncope is an important manifestation of VSA and is caused by ventricular tachyar-rhythmias or bradycardia due to transient conduction disturbances. It is commonly preceded by anginal pain, although not in all cases [70]. The development of arrhythmias is not related to the frequency of angina and concurs with symptomatic as well as asymptomatic myocardial ischemia [20, 21]. More importantly, sudden cardiac death can ensue as a result of coronary artery spasm [71, 72], even in patients with silent myocardial ischemia [21, 22]. In a subgroup of survivors of OHCA, coronary spasm and silent myocardial ischemia were identified as a likely cause of their fatal arrhythmias [21, 22]. Additionally, in the current era, a substantial portion of patients with OHCA survived without neurological deficits by the contribution of increasing use of bystander cardiopulmonary resuscitation, implantable cardioverter-defibrillator (ICD), and hypothermia therapy and a certain number of them have coronary spasm [73]. VSA patients who survived OHCA are particularly high-risk population even in the current era with long-acting CCBs [36]. Implantation of an ICD with medication for VSA might be appropriate for this high-risk population [74]. Recently, we examined the long-term prognosis of patients with OHCA classified based on the results of the dual induction tests for coronary artery spasm and lethal ventricular arrhythmias and evaluated the necessity of ICD by the underlying mechanisms involved (Fig. 1.4) [75]. We found that among OHCA survivors without structural heart disease, provokable coronary spasm and ventricular arrhythmias are common and can be seen in Brugada syndrome (Fig. 1.5a). Then, coronary spasm alone without Brugada syndrome who are treated by CCBs may be a low-risk group (Fig. 1.5b), indicating that ICD may not be essential for OHCA survivors in this low-risk group [75].

1.6   Racial Difference in Vasospastic Angina

For decades, many researchers considered that there may be a racial difference in the prevalence of coronary artery spasm and VSA [76]. For example, variant angina appears to be relatively common in Japan [76]. However, there have been very few studies to systematically examine possible ethnic differences in clinical characteristics and long-term prognosis of VSA patients [59]. Recently, the JCSA conducted

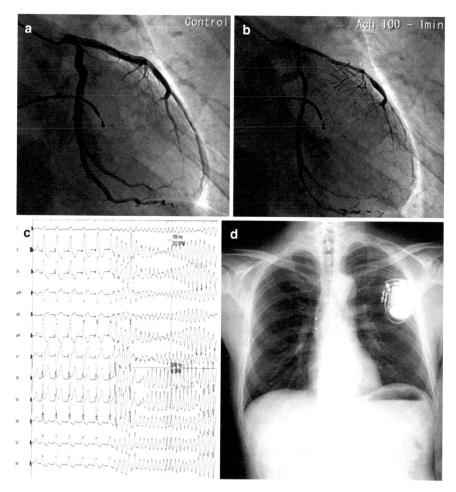

Fig. 1.4 A representative case in the group with both coronary spasm and idiopathic ventricular fibrillation by the dual induction tests. (**a**) Coronary angiogram before spasm provocation test. (**b**) Coronary artery spasm induced by intracoronary acetylcholine. (**c**) Ventricular fibrillation induced by electrophysiological study. (**d**) Subsequent implantation of implantable cardioverter-defibrillator. (Reproduced from Komatsu et al. [75])

an international, prospective, and multicenter registry study, in which a total of 1457 VSA patients (Japanese/Caucasians, 1339/118) were enrolled based on the same diagnostic criteria [77]. Compared with Caucasian patients, Japanese patients were characterized by higher proportions of males (68 vs. 51%) and smoking history (60 vs. 49%). Japanese patients more often had angina especially during the night and early morning hours, compared with Caucasians. Ninety-five percent of Japanese and 84% of Caucasian patients underwent pharmacological provocation test.

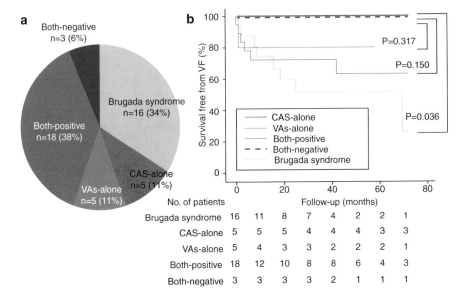

Fig. 1.5 Classification of OHCA survivors when analyzing the patients with Brugada syndrome as a separate group. (**a**) Distribution of patients when the patients with Brugada syndrome were separated as a different group. (**b**) Kaplan–Meier curves for sudden cardiac death by the groups classified by the presence or absence of Brugada syndrome and the dual induction tests. (Reproduced from Komatsu et al. [75])

Importantly, there were no significant differences in the patterns of coronary spasm, with diffuse spasm most frequently noted in both ethnicities. The prescription rate of CCBs was higher in Japanese (96 vs. 86%), whereas the uses of nitrates (46 vs. 59%), statins (43 vs. 65%), renin-angiotensin-system inhibitors (27 vs. 51%), and β-blockers (10 vs. 24%) were more common in Caucasian patients. Survival rate free from MACE was slightly but significantly higher in Japanese than in Caucasians (86.7 vs. 76.6% at 5 years, $P < 0.001$), whereas that free from the hard MACE endpoint was similar (96.5 vs. 97.7%, $P = 0.66$) (Fig. 1.6). Notably, multivariable analysis revealed that the JCSA risk score well correlated with MACE rates not only in Japanese but also in Caucasian patients. These results indicate that there are ethnic differences in clinical profiles and long-term prognosis of contemporary VSA patients [77].

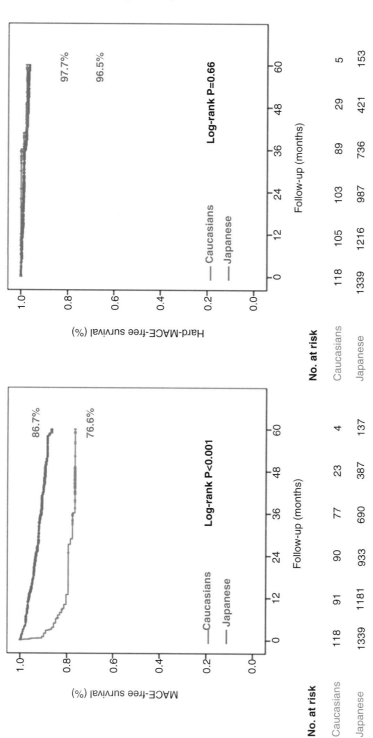

Fig. 1.6 Clinical outcomes of the contemporary Japanese and Caucasians VSA patients. (**a**) Kaplan–Meier curves by ethnics for MACE in VSA patients. MACE included cardiac death, nonfatal myocardial infarction, hospitalization for heart failure and unstable angina pectoris, appropriate ICD shocks, and VT/VF in the patients without ICD. (**b**) Kaplan–Meier curves by ethnics for hard-MACE in VSA patients. Hard-MACE included cardiac death, nonfatal myocardial infarction, VT/VF, and appropriate ICD shocks. (Reproduced from Sato et al. [77])

References

1. Friedberg CK. Some comments and reflections on changing interests and new developments in angina pectoris. Circulation. 1972;46(6):1037–47. https://doi.org/10.1161/01.cir.46.6.1037.
2. Prinzmetal M, Kennamer R, Merliss R, Wada T, Bor N. Angina pectoris. I. A variant form of angina pectoris; preliminary report. Am J Med. 1959;27:375–88. https://doi.org/10.1016/0002-9343(59)90003-8.
3. Gensini GG, Di Giorgi S, Murad-Netto S, Black A. Arteriographic demonstration of coronary artery spasm and its release after the use of a vasodilator in a case of angina pectoris and in the experimental animal. Angiology. 1962;13:550–3. https://doi.org/10.1177/000331976201301202.
4. Yasue H, Touyama M, Shimamoto M, Kato H, Tanaka S. Role of autonomic nervous system in the pathogenesis of Prinzmetal's variant form of angina. Circulation. 1974;50(3):534–9. https://doi.org/10.1161/01.cir.50.3.534.
5. Yasue H, Touyama M, Kato H, Tanaka S, Akiyama F. Prinzmetal's variant form of angina as a manifestation of alpha-adrenergic receptor-mediated coronary artery spasm: documentation by coronary arteriography. Am Heart J. 1976;91(2):148–55. https://doi.org/10.1016/s0002-8703(76)80568-6.
6. Endo M, Hirosawa K, Kaneko N, Hase K, Inoue Y. Prinzmetal's variant angina. Coronary arteriogram and left ventriculogram during angina attack induced by methacholine. N Engl J Med. 1976;294(5):252–5. https://doi.org/10.1056/NEJM197601292940505.
7. Yasue H, Omote S, Takizawa A, Masao N, Hyon H, Nishida S, Horie M. Comparison of coronary arteriographic findings during angina pectoris associated with S-T elevation or depression. Am J Cardiol. 1981;47(3):539–46. https://doi.org/10.1016/0002-9149(81)90536-1.
8. Takeshita A, Koiwaya Y, Nakamura M, Yamamoto K, Torii S. Immediate appearance of coronary collaterals during ergonovine-induced arterial spasm. Chest. 1982;82(3):319–22. https://doi.org/10.1378/chest.82.3.319.
9. Maseri A, Pesola A, Marzilli M, Severi S, Parodi O, L'Abbate A, Ballestra M, Maltinti G, De Nes M, Biagini A. Coronary vasospasm in angina pectoris. Lancet. 1977;1(8014):713–7. https://doi.org/10.1016/s0140-6736(77)92164-x.
10. Maseri A, Beltrame JF, Shimokawa H. Role of coronary vasoconstriction in ischemic heart disease and search for novel therapeutic targets. Circ J. 2009;73(3):394–403. https://doi.org/10.1253/circj.cj-09-0033.
11. Yasue H, Omote S, Takizawa A, Nagao M, Miwa K, Tanaka S. Circadian variation of exercise capacity in patients with Prinzmetal's variant angina: role of exercise-induced coronary arterial spasm. Circulation. 1979;59(5):938–48. https://doi.org/10.1161/01.cir.59.5.938.
12. Specchia G, de Servi S, Falcone C, Bramucci E, Angoli L, Mussini A, Marinoni P, Montemartini C, Bobba P. Coronary arterial spasm as a cause of exercise-induced ST-segment elevation in patients with variant angina. Circulation. 1979;59(5):948–54. https://doi.org/10.1161/01.cir.59.5.948.
13. Boden WE, Bough EW, Korr KS, Benham I, Gheorghiade M, Caputi A, Shulman S. Exercise-induced coronary spasm with S-T segment depression and normal coronary arteriography. Am J Cardiol. 1981;48(1):193–7. https://doi.org/10.1016/0002-9149(81)90591-9.
14. Kaski JC, Crea F, Meran D, Rodriguez L, Araujo L, Chierchia S, Davies G, Maseri A. Local coronary supersensitivity to diverse vasoconstrictive stimuli in patients with variant angina. Circulation. 1986;74(6):1255–65. https://doi.org/10.1161/01.cir.74.6.1255.
15. Waters DD, Miller DD, Bouchard A, Bosch X, Theroux P. Circadian variation in variant angina. Am J Cardiol. 1984;54(1):61–4. https://doi.org/10.1016/0002-9149(84)90304-7.
16. Takusagawa M, Komori S, Umetani K, Ishihara T, Sawanobori T, Kohno I, Sano S, Yin D, Ijiri H, Tamura K. Alterations of autonomic nervous activity in recurrence of variant angina. Heart. 1999;82(1):75–81. https://doi.org/10.1136/hrt.82.1.75.

17. Lanza GA, Pedrotti P, Pasceri V, Lucente M, Crea F, Maseri A. Autonomic changes associated with spontaneous coronary spasm in patients with variant angina. J Am Coll Cardiol. 1996;28(5):1249–56. https://doi.org/10.1016/S0735-1097(96)00309-9.
18. Kawano H, Motoyama T, Yasue H, Hirai N, Waly HM, Kugiyama K, Ogawa H. Endothelial function fluctuates with diurnal variation in the frequency of ischemic episodes in patients with variant angina. J Am Coll Cardiol. 2002;40(2):266–70. https://doi.org/10.1016/s0735-1097(02)01956-3.
19. Nihei T, Takahashi J, Tsuburaya R, Ito Y, Shiroto T, Hao K, Takagi Y, Matsumoto Y, Nakayama M, Miyata S, Sakata Y, Ito K, Shimokawa H. Circadian variation of Rho-kinase activity in circulating leukocytes of patients with vasospastic angina. Circ J. 2014;78(5):1183–90. https://doi.org/10.1253/circj.cj-13-1458.
20. Araki H, Koiwaya Y, Nakagaki O, Nakamura M. Diurnal distribution of ST-segment elevation and related arrhythmias in patients with variant angina: a study by ambulatory ECG monitoring. Circulation. 1983;67(5):995–1000. https://doi.org/10.1161/01.cir.67.5.995.
21. Myerburg RJ, Kessler KM, Mallon SM, Cox MM, deMarchena E, Interian A Jr, Castellanos A. Life-threatening ventricular arrhythmias in patients with silent myocardial ischemia due to coronary-artery spasm. N Engl J Med. 1992;326(22):1451–5. https://doi.org/10.1056/NEJM199205283262202.
22. Chevalier P, Dacosta A, Defaye P, Chalvidan T, Bonnefoy E, Kirkorian G, Isaaz K, Denis B, Touboul P. Arrhythmic cardiac arrest due to isolated coronary artery spasm: long-term outcome of seven resuscitated patients. J Am Coll Cardiol. 1998;31(1):57–61. https://doi.org/10.1016/s0735-1097(97)00442-7.
23. Oliva PB, Breckinridge JC. Arteriographic evidence of coronary arterial spasm in acute myocardial infarction. Circulation. 1977;56(3):366–74. https://doi.org/10.1161/01.cir.56.3.366.
24. Maseri A, L'Abbate A, Baroldi G, Chierchia S, Marzilli M, Ballestra AM, Severi S, Parodi O, Biagini A, Distante A, Pesola A. Coronary vasospasm as a possible cause of myocardial infarction. A conclusion derived from the study of "preinfarction" angina. N Engl J Med. 1978;299(23):1271–7. https://doi.org/10.1056/NEJM197812072992303.
25. Fukai T, Koyanagi S, Takeshita A. Role of coronary vasospasm in the pathogenesis of myocardial infarction: study in patients with no significant coronary stenosis. Am Heart J. 1993;126(6):1305–11. https://doi.org/10.1016/0002-8703(93)90527-g.
26. Ong P, Athanasiadis A, Hill S, Vogelsberg H, Voehringer M, Sechtem U. Coronary artery spasm as a frequent cause of acute coronary syndrome: the CASPAR (coronary artery spasm in patients with acute coronary syndrome) study. J Am Coll Cardiol. 2008;52(7):523–7. https://doi.org/10.1016/j.jacc.2008.04.050.
27. Mueller HS, Cohen LS, Braunwald E, Forman S, Feit F, Ross A, Schweiger M, Cabin H, Davison R, Miller D. Predictors of early morbidity and mortality after thrombolytic therapy of acute myocardial infarction. Analyses of patient subgroups in the thrombolysis in myocardial infarction (TIMI) trial, phase II. Circulation. 1992;85(4):1254–64. https://doi.org/10.1161/01.cir.85.4.1254.
28. Nakamura M, Koiwaya Y. Effect of diltiazem on recurrent spontaneous angina after acute myocardial infarction. Circ Res. 1983;52(2 Pt 2):I158–62.
29. Koiwaya Y, Torii S, Takeshita A, Nakagaki O, Nakamura M. Postinfarction angina caused by coronary arterial spasm. Circulation. 1982;65(2):275–80. https://doi.org/10.1161/01.cir.65.2.275.
30. Wakabayashi K, Suzuki H, Honda Y, Wakatsuki D, Kawachi K, Ota K, Koba S, Shimizu N, Asano F, Sato T, Takeyama Y. Provoked coronary spasm predicts adverse outcome in patients with acute myocardial infarction: a novel predictor of prognosis after acute myocardial infarction. J Am Coll Cardiol. 2008;52(7):518–22. https://doi.org/10.1016/j.jacc.2008.01.076.
31. Ogawa H, Suefuji H, Soejima H, Nishiyama K, Misumi K, Takazoe K, Miyamoto S, Kajikawa I, Sumida H, Sakamoto T, Yoshimura M, Kugiyama K, Yasue H, Matsuo K. Increased blood vascular endothelial growth factor levels in patients with acute myocardial infarction. Cardiology. 2000;93(1–2):93–9. https://doi.org/10.1159/000007008.

32. Sueda S, Kohno H, Fukuda H, Uraoka T. Did the widespread use of long-acting calcium antagonists decrease the occurrence of variant angina? Chest. 2003;124(6):2074–8. https://doi.org/10.1378/chest.124.6.2074.
33. Bertrand ME, LaBlanche JM, Tilmant PY, Thieuleux FA, Delforge MR, Carre AG, Asseman P, Berzin B, Libersa C, Laurent JM. Frequency of provoked coronary arterial spasm in 1089 consecutive patients undergoing coronary arteriography. Circulation. 1982;65(7):1299–306. https://doi.org/10.1161/01.cir.65.7.1299.
34. Sueda S, Ochi N, Kawada H, Matsuda S, Hayashi Y, Tsuruoka T, Uraoka T. Frequency of provoked coronary vasospasm in patients undergoing coronary arteriography with spasm provocation test of acetylcholine. Am J Cardiol. 1999;83(8):1186–90. https://doi.org/10.1016/s0002-9149(99)00057-0.
35. Pristipino C, Beltrame JF, Finocchiaro ML, Hattori R, Fujita M, Mongiardo R, Cianflone D, Sanna T, Sasayama S, Maseri A. Major racial differences in coronary constrictor response between Japanese and Caucasians with recent myocardial infarction. Circulation. 2000;101(10):1102–8. https://doi.org/10.1161/01.cir.101.10.1102.
36. Takagi Y, Yasuda S, Tsunoda R, Ogata Y, Seki A, Sumiyoshi T, Matsui M, Goto T, Tanabe Y, Sueda S, Sato T, Ogawa H, Kubo N, Momomura S, Ogawa H, Shimokawa H. Clinical characteristics and long-term prognosis of vasospastic angina patients who survived out-of-hospital cardiac arrest: multicenter registry study of the Japanese Coronary Spasm Association. Circ Arrhythm Electrophysiol. 2011;4(3):295–302. https://doi.org/10.1161/CIRCEP.110.959809.
37. Ong P, Athanasiadis A, Borgulya G, Mahrholdt H, Kaski JC, Sechtem U. High prevalence of a pathological response to acetylcholine testing in patients with stable angina pectoris and unobstructed coronary arteries. The ACOVA study (Abnormal COronary VAsomotion in patients with stable angina and unobstructed coronary arteries). J Am Coll Cardiol. 2012;59(7):655–62. https://doi.org/10.1016/j.jacc.2011.11.015.
38. Montone RA, Niccoli G, Fracassi F, Russo M, Gurgoglione F, Camma G, Lanza GA, Crea F. Patients with acute myocardial infarction and non-obstructive coronary arteries: safety and prognostic relevance of invasive coronary provocative tests. Eur Heart J. 2018;39(2):91–8. https://doi.org/10.1093/eurheartj/ehx667.
39. Hung MJ, Cherng WJ, Cheng CW, Li LF. Comparison of serum levels of inflammatory markers in patients with coronary vasospasm without significant fixed coronary artery disease versus patients with stable angina pectoris and acute coronary syndromes with significant fixed coronary artery disease. Am J Cardiol. 2006;97(10):1429–34. https://doi.org/10.1016/j.amjcard.2005.12.035.
40. Hung MJ, Cheng CW, Yang NI, Hung MY, Cherng WJ. Coronary vasospasm-induced acute coronary syndrome complicated by life-threatening cardiac arrhythmias in patients without hemodynamically significant coronary artery disease. Int J Cardiol. 2007;117(1):37–44. https://doi.org/10.1016/j.ijcard.2006.03.055.
41. Ong P, Athanasiadis A, Borgulya G, Vokshi I, Bastiaenen R, Kubik S, Hill S, Schaufele T, Mahrholdt H, Kaski JC, Sechtem U. Clinical usefulness, angiographic characteristics, and safety evaluation of intracoronary acetylcholine provocation testing among 921 consecutive white patients with unobstructed coronary arteries. Circulation. 2014;129(17):1723–30. https://doi.org/10.1161/CIRCULATIONAHA.113.004096.
42. Takaoka K, Yoshimura M, Ogawa H, Kugiyama K, Nakayama M, Shimasaki Y, Mizuno Y, Sakamoto T, Yasue H. Comparison of the risk factors for coronary artery spasm with those for organic stenosis in a Japanese population: role of cigarette smoking. Int J Cardiol. 2000;72(2):121–6. https://doi.org/10.1016/s0167-5273(99)00172-2.
43. Hung MJ, Cherng WJ, Yang NI, Cheng CW, Li LF. Relation of high-sensitivity C-reactive protein level with coronary vasospastic angina pectoris in patients without hemodynamically significant coronary artery disease. Am J Cardiol. 2005;96(11):1484–90. https://doi.org/10.1016/j.amjcard.2005.07.055.
44. Miwa K, Makita T, Ishii K, Okuda N, Taniguchi A. High remnant lipoprotein levels in patients with variant angina. Clin Cardiol. 2004;27(6):338–42. https://doi.org/10.1002/clc.4960270608.

45. Oi K, Shimokawa H, Hiroki J, Uwatoku T, Abe K, Matsumoto Y, Nakajima Y, Nakajima K, Takeischi S, Takeshita A. Remnant lipoproteins from patients with sudden cardiac death enhance coronary vasospastic activity through upregulation of Rho-kinase. Arterioscler Thromb Vasc Biol. 2004;24(5):918–22. https://doi.org/10.1161/01.ATV.0000126678.93747.80.

46. Yasue H, Kugiyama K. Coronary spasm: clinical features and pathogenesis. Intern Med. 1997;36(11):760–5. https://doi.org/10.2169/internalmedicine.36.760.

47. Sugiishi M, Takatsu F. Cigarette smoking is a major risk factor for coronary spasm. Circulation. 1993;87(1):76–9. https://doi.org/10.1161/01.cir.87.1.76.

48. Nobuyoshi M, Abe M, Nosaka H, Kimura T, Yokoi H, Hamasaki N, Shindo T, Kimura K, Nakamura T, Nakagawa Y. Statistical analysis of clinical risk factors for coronary artery spasm: identification of the most important determinant. Am Heart J. 1992;124(1):32–8. https://doi.org/10.1016/0002-8703(92)90917-k.

49. Caralis DG, Deligonul U, Kern MJ, Cohen JD. Smoking is a risk factor for coronary spasm in young women. Circulation. 1992;85(3):905–9. https://doi.org/10.1161/01.cir.85.3.905.

50. Hung MY, Hsu KH, Hung MJ, Cheng CW, Kuo LT, Cherng WJ. Interaction between cigarette smoking and high-sensitivity C-reactive protein in the development of coronary vasospasm in patients without hemodynamically significant coronary artery disease. Am J Med Sci. 2009;338(6):440–6. https://doi.org/10.1097/MAJ.0b013e3181b9147f.

51. Kawana A, Takahashi J, Takagi Y, Yasuda S, Sakata Y, Tsunoda R, Ogata Y, Seki A, Sumiyoshi T, Matsui M, Goto T, Tanabe Y, Sueda S, Kubo N, Momomura S, Ogawa H, Shimokawa H. Gender differences in the clinical characteristics and outcomes of patients with vasospastic angina--a report from the Japanese Coronary Spasm Association. Circ J. 2013;77(5):1267–74. https://doi.org/10.1253/circj.cj-12-1486.

52. Shimokawa H. 2014 Williams Harvey lecture: importance of coronary vasomotion abnormalities-from bench to bedside. Eur Heart J. 2014;35(45):3180–93. https://doi.org/10.1093/eurheartj/ehu427.

53. Hiroki J, Shimokawa H, Mukai Y, Ichiki T, Takeshita A. Divergent effects of estrogen and nicotine on Rho-kinase expression in human coronary vascular smooth muscle cells. Biochem Biophys Res Commun. 2005;326(1):154–9. https://doi.org/10.1016/j.bbrc.2004.11.011.

54. Miwa K, Fujita M, Miyagi Y. Beneficial effects of smoking cessation on the short-term prognosis for variant angina--validation of the smoking status by urinary cotinine measurements. Int J Cardiol. 1994;44(2):151–6. https://doi.org/10.1016/0167-5273(94)90019-1.

55. Shinozaki K, Suzuki M, Ikebuchi M, Takaki H, Hara Y, Tsushima M, Harano Y. Insulin resistance associated with compensatory hyperinsulinemia as an independent risk factor for vasospastic angina. Circulation. 1995;92(7):1749–57. https://doi.org/10.1161/01.cir.92.7.1749.

56. Miwa K, Fujita M, Miyagi Y, Inoue H, Sasayama S. High-density lipoprotein cholesterol level and smoking modify the prognosis of patients with coronary vasospasm. Clin Cardiol. 1995;18(5):267–72. https://doi.org/10.1002/clc.4960180508.

57. Itoh T, Mizuno Y, Harada E, Yoshimura M, Ogawa H, Yasue H. Coronary spasm is associated with chronic low-grade inflammation. Circ J. 2007;71(7):1074–8. https://doi.org/10.1253/circj.71.1074.

58. Yasue H, Mizuno Y, Harada E, Itoh T, Nakagawa H, Nakayama M, Ogawa H, Tayama S, Honda T, Hokimoto S, Ohshima S, Hokamura Y, Kugiyama K, Horie M, Yoshimura M, Harada M, Uemura S, Saito Y. Effects of a 3-hydroxy-3-methylglutaryl coenzyme A reductase inhibitor, fluvastatin, on coronary spasm after withdrawal of calcium-channel blockers. J Am Coll Cardiol. 2008;51(18):1742–8. https://doi.org/10.1016/j.jacc.2007.12.049.

59. Shimokawa H, Nagasawa K, Irie T, Egashira S, Egashira K, Sagara T, Kikuchi Y, Nakamura M. Clinical characteristics and long-term prognosis of patients with variant angina. A comparative study between western and Japanese populations. Int J Cardiol. 1988;18(3):331–49. https://doi.org/10.1016/0167-5273(88)90052-6.

60. Yasue H, Takizawa A, Nagao M, Nishida S, Horie M, Kubota J, Omote S, Takaoka K, Okumura K. Long-term prognosis for patients with variant angina and influential factors. Circulation. 1988;78(1):1–9. https://doi.org/10.1161/01.cir.78.1.1.

61. Walling A, Waters DD, Miller DD, Roy D, Pelletier GB, Theroux P. Long-term prognosis of patients with variant angina. Circulation. 1987;76(5):990–7. https://doi.org/10.1161/01. cir.76.5.990.

62. Ueshima H. Explanation for the Japanese paradox: prevention of increase in coronary heart disease and reduction in stroke. J Atheroscler Thromb. 2007;14(6):278–86. https://doi. org/10.5551/jat.e529.

63. Ong P, Athanasiadis A, Borgulya G, Voehringer M, Sechtem U. 3-year follow-up of patients with coronary artery spasm as cause of acute coronary syndrome: the CASPAR (coronary artery spasm in patients with acute coronary syndrome) study follow-up. J Am Coll Cardiol. 2011;57(2):147–52. https://doi.org/10.1016/j.jacc.2010.08.626.

64. Lette J, Gagnon RM, Lemire JG, Morissette M. Rebound of vasospastic angina after cessation of long-term treatment with nifedipine. Can Med Assoc J. 1984;130(9):1169–71. 74

65. Waters DD, Miller DD, Szlachcic J, Bouchard A, Methe M, Kreeft J, Theroux P. Factors influencing the long-term prognosis of treated patients with variant angina. Circulation. 1983;68(2):258–65. https://doi.org/10.1161/01.cir.68.2.258.

66. Mark DB, Califf RM, Morris KG, Harrell FE Jr, Pryor DB, Hlatky MA, Lee KL, Rosati RA. Clinical characteristics and long-term survival of patients with variant angina. Circulation. 1984;69(5):880–8. https://doi.org/10.1161/01.cir.69.5.880.

67. Lanza GA, Sestito A, Sgueglia GA, Infusino F, Manolfi M, Crea F, Maseri A. Current clinical features, diagnostic assessment and prognostic determinants of patients with variant angina. Int J Cardiol. 2007;118(1):41–7. https://doi.org/10.1016/j.ijcard.2006.06.016.

68. Takagi Y, Yasuda S, Takahashi J, Tsunoda R, Ogata Y, Seki A, Sumiyoshi T, Matsui M, Goto T, Tanabe Y, Sueda S, Kubo N, Momomura S, Ogawa H, Shimokawa H. Clinical implications of provocation tests for coronary artery spasm: safety, arrhythmic complications, and prognostic impact: multicentre registry study of the Japanese Coronary Spasm Association. Eur Heart J. 2013;34(4):258–67. https://doi.org/10.1093/eurheartj/ehs199.

69. Takagi Y, Takahashi J, Yasuda S, Miyata S, Tsunoda R, Ogata Y, Seki A, Sumiyoshi T, Matsui M, Goto T, Tanabe Y, Sueda S, Kubo N, Momomura S, Ogawa H, Shimokawa H. Prognostic stratification of patients with vasospastic angina: a comprehensive clinical risk score developed by the Japanese Coronary Spasm Association. J Am Coll Cardiol. 2013;62(13):1144–53. https://doi.org/10.1016/j.jacc.2013.07.018.

70. Maseri A, Chierchia S. Coronary artery spasm: demonstration, definition, diagnosis, and consequences. Prog Cardiovasc Dis. 1982;25(3):169–92. https://doi. org/10.1016/0033-0620(82)90015-9.

71. Roberts WC, Curry RC Jr, Isner JM, Waller BF, McManus BM, Mariani-Costantini R, Ross AM. Sudden death in Prinzmetal's angina with coronary spasm documented by angiography. Analysis of three necropsy patients. Am J Cardiol. 1982;50(1):203–10. https://doi. org/10.1016/0002-9149(82)90030-3.

72. Miller DD, Waters DD, Szlachcic J, Theroux P. Clinical characteristics associated with sudden death in patients with variant angina. Circulation. 1982;66(3):588–92. https://doi. org/10.1161/01.cir.66.3.588.

73. Takagi Y, Yasuda S, Takahashi J, Takeda M, Nakayama M, Ito K, Hirose M, Wakayama Y, Fukuda K, Shimokawa H. Importance of dual induction tests for coronary vasospasm and ventricular fibrillation in patients surviving out-of-hospital cardiac arrest. Circ J. 2009;73(4):767–9. https://doi.org/10.1253/circj.cj-09-0061.

74. Matsue Y, Suzuki M, Nishizaki M, Hojo R, Hashimoto Y, Sakurada H. Clinical implications of an implantable cardioverter-defibrillator in patients with vasospastic angina and lethal ventricular arrhythmia. J Am Coll Cardiol. 2012;60(10):908–13. https://doi.org/10.1016/j. jacc.2012.03.070.

75. Komatsu M, Takahashi J, Fukuda K, Takagi Y, Shiroto T, Nakano M, Kondo M, Tsuburaya R, Hao K, Nishimiya K, Nihei T, Matsumoto Y, Ito K, Sakata Y, Miyata S, Shimokawa H. Usefulness of testing for coronary artery spasm and programmed ventricular stimulation in

survivors of out-of-hospital cardiac arrest. Circ Arrhythm Electrophysiol. 2016;9(9):e003798. https://doi.org/10.1161/CIRCEP.115.003798.

76. Beltrame JF, Sasayama S, Maseri A. Racial heterogeneity in coronary artery vasomotor reactivity: differences between Japanese and Caucasian patients. J Am Coll Cardiol. 1999;33(6):1442–52. https://doi.org/10.1016/s0735-1097(99)00073-x.

77. Sato K, Takahashi J, Odaka Y, Suda A, Sueda S, Teragawa H, Ishii K, Kiyooka T, Hirayama A, Sumiyoshi T, Tanabe Y, Kimura K, Kaikita K, Ong P, Sechtem U, Camici PG, Kaski JC, Crea F, Beltrame JF, Shimokawa H. Clinical characteristics and long-term prognosis of contemporary patients with vasospastic angina: ethnic differences detected in an international comparative study. Int J Cardiol. 2019;291:13–8. https://doi.org/10.1016/j.ijcard.2019.02.038.

Chapter 2
Pathophysiology and Molecular Mechanisms of Coronary Artery Spasm

Kimio Satoh and Hiroaki Shimokawa

Abstract Rho-kinase plays a central role in the pathogenesis of coronary artery spasm caused by vascular smooth muscle cell (VSMC) hypercontraction. Rho-kinase belongs to the family of serine/threonine kinases and is an important downstream effector of the small GTP-binding protein RhoA. Two isoforms of Rho-kinase, ROCK1 and ROCK2, have different functions with ROCK1 for circulating inflammatory cells and ROCK2 for vascular smooth muscle cells. The RhoA/Rho-kinase pathway plays an important role in many cellular functions, including contraction, motility, proliferation, and apoptosis, leading to the development of cardiovascular diseases. In addition to vasospasm, important roles of Rho-kinase in vivo have been demonstrated in the pathogenesis of arteriosclerosis, ischemia/reperfusion injury, hypertension, pulmonary hypertension, stroke, and heart failure. Furthermore, the beneficial effects of fasudil, a selective Rho-kinase inhibitor, have been demonstrated for the treatment of several cardiovascular diseases in animals and humans. Thus, the Rho-kinase pathway is an important new therapeutic target in vasospasm and other cardiovascular diseases.

Keywords Vasospasm · Rho-kinase · Cardiovascular disease · Oxidative stress · Small G proteins

K. Satoh · H. Shimokawa (✉)
Department of Cardiovascular Medicine, Tohoku University Graduate School of Medicine, Sendai, Miyagi, Japan
e-mail: shimo@cardio.med.tohoku.ac.jp

© Springer Nature Singapore Pte Ltd. 2021
H. Shimokawa (ed.), *Coronary Vasomotion Abnormalities*,
https://doi.org/10.1007/978-981-15-7594-5_2

2.1 Development of Animal Models of Coronary Artery Spasm and Identification of Important Pathogenetic Roles of Rho-Kinase

Rho-kinase activation plays a central role in the pathogenesis of coronary artery spasm caused by vascular smooth muscle cell (VSMC) hypercontraction. In an animal model in pigs in vivo, we examined whether atherosclerotic coronary lesion, induced by a combination of balloon endothelium removal and high-cholesterol feeding, exhibits hyperresponsiveness to vasoconstrictor agents [1]. Importantly, intracoronary administration of serotonin induced coronary artery spasm at the atherosclerotic lesion, and there was a close topological correlation between the spastic site and atherosclerotic lesion (Fig. 2.1a, b) [1]. This is the first experimental evidence for the close relationship between coronary artery spasm and coronary atherosclerosis [1]. Next, we further examined whether chronic adventitial inflammation could cause vasospastic activity of the coronary artery without endothelium removal in pigs. Two weeks after the adventitial application of interleukin-1β (IL-1β), coronary angiography showed the development of mild stenotic lesion, where intracoronary administration of serotonin repeatedly caused coronary spasm (Fig. 2.1c) [2]. Histological examination showed adventitial accumulation of inflammatory cells, mild neointimal formation, and a marked reduction in vascular cross-sectional area (Fig. 2.1d) [2]. These results provided the first experimental evidence for the role of adventitial inflammation in the pathogenesis of coronary artery spasm. Delayed cerebral ischemia due to cerebral vasospasm remains a major cause of morbidity in patients with subarachnoid hemorrhage (SAH). It has been demonstrated that Rho-kinase is substantially involved in the pathogenesis of cerebral vasospasm after SAH [3]. Coronary artery spasm plays an important role in variant angina, myocardial infarction, and sudden cardiac death [4]. It was demonstrated that elevated serum level of cortisol, one of the important stress hormones, causes coronary hyperreactivity through activation of Rho-kinase in pigs in vivo [5]. The activity and the expression of ROCKs are enhanced at the inflammatory/arteriosclerotic coronary lesions [6]. Accumulating evidence indicates that Rho-kinase plays a crucial role in the pathogenesis of coronary artery spasm. Intracoronary administration of fasudil [7] and of hydroxyfasudil [8] inhibited coronary spasm in pigs in vivo [2]. We have demonstrated that fasudil is effective in preventing coronary spasm and resultant myocardial ischemia in patients with vasospastic angina [9]. Thus, fasudil is useful for the treatment of ischemic coronary syndromes caused by coronary artery spasm. Fasudil is also effective in treating patients with microvascular angina [10]. The clinical trials for the effects of fasudil in Japanese patients with stable-effort angina demonstrated that the long-term oral treatment with the Rho-kinase inhibitor is effective in ameliorating exercise tolerance in those patients [11]. We also have recently demonstrated that Rho-kinase activity in circulating neutrophils is an useful biomarker for the diagnosis and disease activity assessment in patients with VSA [12].

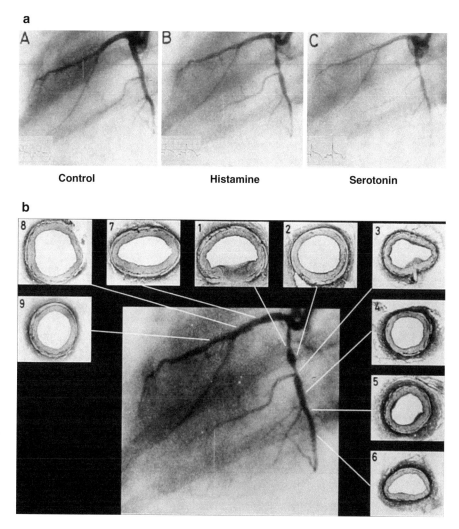

Fig. 2.1 Coronary artery spasm induced in two porcine models in vivo. (**a**, **b**) Coronary artery spasm was induced in atherosclerotic miniature pigs induced by balloon endothelial injury and high-cholesterol feeding (**a**), where topological correlation was noted between the spastic sites and the early atherosclerotic lesions (**b**). (**c**, **d**) Coronary artery spasm was induced in pigs with adventitial inflammation (**c**), where intimal thickening and negative remodeling were noted (**d**). (Reproduced from Shimokawa et al. [1, 2])

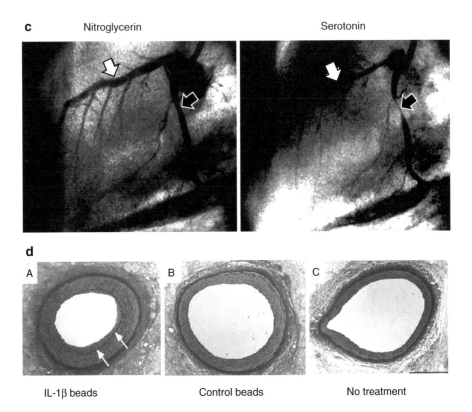

Fig. 2.1 (continued)

2.2   The Rho/Rho-Kinase System in Vascular Contraction

Rho-kinase belongs to the family of serine/threonine kinases and is an important downstream effector of the small GTP-binding protein RhoA. The Rho family of small G proteins comprises 20 members of ubiquitously expressed proteins in mammals, including RhoA, Rac1, and Cdc42 [13–15]. Among them, RhoA is the best-characterized protein that acts as a molecular switch that cycles between an inactive GDP-bound and an active GTP-bound conformation interacting with downstream targets to elicit a variety of cellular responses (Fig. 2.2) [16]. The activity of RhoA is controlled by the guanine nucleotide exchange factors (GEFs) that catalyze exchange of GDP for GTP [17]. In contrast, GTPase activating proteins (GAPs) stimulate the intrinsic GTPase activity and inactivate RhoA [18]. Additionally, it has been demonstrated that guanine nucleotide dissociation inhibitors (GDIs) block spontaneous RhoA activation (Fig. 2.2) [19].

In 1996, Rho-kinase (Rho-kinase α/ROCK 2/ROKα and Rho-kinase β/ROCK 1/ROKβ) was identified as the effector of Rho (Fig. 2.2) [20–22]. Phosphorylation of

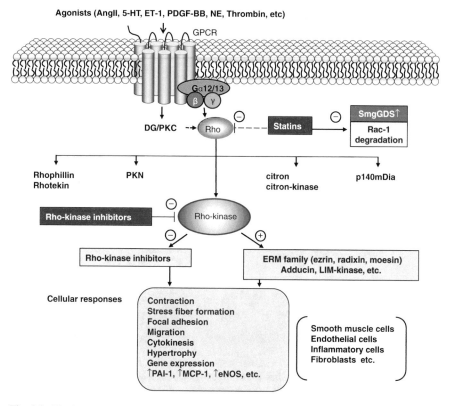

Fig. 2.2 The important roles of Rho/Rho-kinase pathway in the pathogenesis of cardiovascular diseases. The Rho/Rho-kinase pathway plays important roles in the pathogenesis of vasospastic disorders as well as atherosclerotic cardiovascular diseases in general. (Reproduced from Shimokawa et al. [27])

myosin light chain (MLC) is a key event in the regulation of VSMC contraction (Fig. 2.3). MLC is phosphorylated by Ca^{2+}-calmodulin-activated MLC kinase (MLCK) and dephosphorylated by MLC phosphatase (MLCP) (Fig. 2.3). Agonists bind to G-protein-coupled receptors and induce contraction by increasing both cytosolic Ca^{2+} concentration and Rho-kinase activity through mediating GEF. The substrates of Rho-kinase have been identified, including MLC, myosin-binding subunit (MBS) or myosin phosphatase target subunit (MYPT-1), ERM family, adducin, PTEN, and LIM-kinases (Figs. 2.2 and 2.3). Rho-kinase enhances MLC phosphorylation through inhibition of MBS of myosin phosphatase and mediate agonists-induced VSMC contraction (Fig. 2.3).

The interaction between endothelial cells (ECs) and VSMCs plays an important role in regulating vascular integrity and vascular homeostasis [23, 24]. ECs release vasoactive factors, such as prostacyclin, nitric oxide (NO) and endothelium-derived hyperpolarizing factor (EDHF), participating in the regulation of vascular tone and arterial resistance [1, 25–27]. It has been demonstrated that both endothelial NO

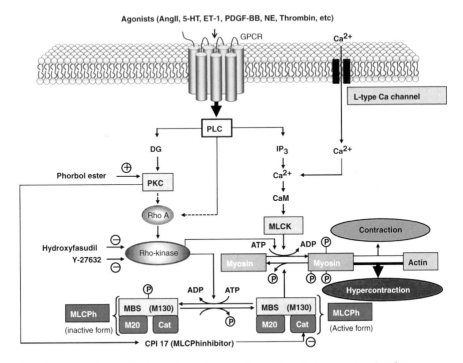

Fig. 2.3 Molecular mechanisms of vascular smooth muscle cells hypercontraction for coronary spasm. The central molecular mechanism of vascular smooth muscle cell hypercontraction for coronary spasm is Rho-kinase-mediated enhancement of myosin light chain phosphorylations through inhibition of myosin light chain phosphatase. (Reproduced from Shimokawa et al. [27])

production and NO-mediated signaling in VSMCs are targets and effectors of the RhoA/Rho-kinase pathway [23, 28]. In ECs, the RhoA/Rho-kinase pathway negatively regulates NO production [29]. In contrast, VSMCs are among the most plastic of all cells in their ability to respond to different stimuli [30–32]. The initial works in our laboratory on the therapeutic importance of Rho-kinase were previously summarized [23, 33]. Since then, a significant progress has been made in our knowledge on the therapeutic importance of Rho-kinase in cardiovascular medicine. In this article, we will briefly review the recent progress in the translational research on the therapeutic importance of the Rho-kinase pathway in cardiovascular medicine.

2.3 Substrates of Rho-Kinase

Rho-kinase is a serine/threonine kinase with a molecular weight of ~160 kDa. Two isoforms of Rho-kinase encoded by 2 different genes have been identified [34–36]. In humans, ROCK1 and ROCK2 genes are located separately on chromosome 18 and chromosome 2, respectively. They are ubiquitously expressed in invertebrates and vertebrates with ROCK1 especially in circulating inflammatory cells and ROCK2 in VSMCs. ROCKs consist of 3 major domains, including a kinase domain in its N-terminal domain, a coiled–coil domain that includes Rho-binding domain in its middle portion, and a putative pleckstrin homology (PH) domain in its C-terminal domain [13]. Rho-kinase activity is enhanced by binding of GTP-bound active form of RhoA [35] (Fig. 2.2). Rho-kinase inhibitors, fasudil [8] and Y-27632 [37], have been developed and they inhibit Rho-kinase activity in a competitive manner with ATP at the Rho-binding site [38]. It has been demonstrated that hydroxyfasudil, a major active metabolite of fasudil, exerts a more specific inhibitory effect on Rho-kinase [8, 39].

Although regulation of Rho-kinase expression has not been fully elucidated, some studies have reported changes in Rho-kinase expression. Functional differences between ROCK1 and ROCK2 have been reported; ROCK1 is specifically cleaved by caspase-3, whereas ROCK2 is cleaved by granzyme B [40, 41]. The small G-protein RhoE specially binds to the N-terminal region of ROCK1 at the kinase domain, whereas the MYPT1 binds specially ROCK2 [42, 43]. RhoE binding to ROCK1 inhibits its activity and prevents RhoA binding to the Rho-binding domain [44]. Both ROCK1 and ROCK2 mRNAs and proteins are upregulated by angiotensin II (AngII) via AT1 receptor stimulation and by interleukin-1β (IL-1β) [45]. A number of Rho-kinase substrates have been identified [46] (Fig. 2.2) and Rho-kinase-mediated substrate phosphorylation causes actin filament formation, organization, and cytoskeleton rearrangement (Fig. 2.2) [47]. The N-terminal regions, upstream of the kinase domains of Rho-kinase, may play a role in determining substrate specificity of the 2 isoforms [47].

The majority of Rho-kinase substrates have been identified in vitro. Thus, ROCK1- and ROCK2-deficient mice have been generated to further elucidate the functions of the ROCK isoforms [48, 49]. Importantly, ROCK1-deficient mice showed the eyelids opened at birth [49], whereas ROCK2-deficient mice placental dysfunction and fetal death [48, 50–52]. Thus, the role of ROCK2, the main isoform in the cardiovascular system, remained to be fully elucidated in vivo. In order to address this point, we have recently developed VSMC-specific ROCK2-deficient mice and found the crucial role of ROCK2 in the development of hypoxia-induced pulmonary hypertension [30].

2.4   Rho-Kinase-Mediated Inflammation and Oxidative Stress

Rho-kinase augments inflammation by inducing pro-inflammatory molecules, including IL-6 [53], monocyte chemoattractant protein (MCP)-1 [54], macrophage migration inhibitory factor (MIF) [55, 56], and sphingosine-1-phosphate (S1P) [57]. In ECs, Rho-kinase downregulates eNOS [58] and substantially activates pro-inflammatory pathways including enhanced expression of adhesion molecules. The expression of Rho-kinase is accelerated by inflammatory stimuli, such as AngII and

IL-1β [45], and by remnant lipoproteins in human coronary VSMCs [59]. Rho-kinase also upregulates NAD(P)H oxidases and augments AngII-induced ROS production [39]. Several growth factors are known to be secreted from VSMC in response to oxidative stress. Rho GTPases including RhoA are key regulators in signaling pathways linked to actin cytoskeletal rearrangement [60]. RhoA plays a central role in vesicular trafficking pathways by controlling organization of actin cytoskeleton. It has been reported that active participation of Rho GTPases is required for secretion. Myosin II is involved in secretory mechanisms as a motor for vesicle transport [61]. Rho-kinase mediates myosin II activation via phosphorylation and inactivation of myosin II light chain phosphatase [20]. Thus, the Rho/Rho-kinase is important for the secretion of inflammatory cytokines and growth factors (Fig. 2.2).

2.5 Rho-Kinase in Vascular Function and Contraction

Rho-kinase has been implicated in the pathogenesis of cardiovascular disease, in part by promoting VSMC proliferation [62–64]. Changes in vascular redox state are a common pathway involved in the pathogenesis of vasospastic angina (VSA), atherosclerosis, aortic aneurysms, and vascular stenosis. Vascular ROS formation can be stimulated by mechanical stretch, pressure overload, shear stress, environmental factors (e.g. hypoxia), and growth factors (e.g. AngII) [65]. Importantly, Rho-kinase is substantially involved in the vascular effects of various vasoactive factors, including AngII [39, 54, 66, 67], thrombin [68, 69], platelet-derived growth factor [70], extracellular nucleotides [71], and urotensin [72] (Fig. 2.2). It has previously been shown that statins enhance eNOS mRNA by cholesterol-independent mechanisms involving inhibition of Rho geranylgeranylation [73]. Rho-kinase plays an important role in mediating various cellular functions, not only VSMC contraction [74, 75] but also actin cytoskeleton organization [76, 77], adhesion, and cytokinesis [33]. Thus, Rho-kinase plays a crucial role in the development of cardiovascular disease through ROS production, inflammation, EC damage, VSMC contraction and proliferation (Figs. 2.2 and 2.3).

2.6 Rho-Kinase in Arteriosclerosis

As mentioned above, Rho-kinase plays a crucial role in the ROS augmentation and vascular inflammation. ROS have been implicated in the pathogenesis of neointima formation in part by promoting VSMC growth [64, 78] and by stimulating pro-inflammatory events [79–81]. Accumulating evidence indicates that Rho-kinase inhibitors have broad pharmacological properties [33, 75, 82]. The beneficial effects of long-term inhibition of Rho-kinase for the treatment of cardiovascular disease have been demonstrated in various animal models, such as coronary artery spasm, arteriosclerosis, restenosis, ischemia/reperfusion injury, hypertension, pulmonary hypertension, stroke, and cardiac hypertrophy/heart failure [33, 75, 82]. Gene transfer of dominant-negative Rho-kinase reduced the neointimal formation in pigs [83]. Long-term treatment with a Rho-kinase inhibitor suppressed neointima formation after vascular injury in vivo [84, 85], MCP-1-induced vascular lesion formation [86], constrictive remodeling [87], in-stent restenosis [88], and the development of cardiac allograft vasculopathy [56] (Fig. 2.2).

Arteriosclerosis is a slowly progressing inflammatory process of the arterial wall that involves the intima, media, and adventitia [33, 75]. Accumulating evidence indicates that Rho-kinase-mediated pathway is substantially involved in EC dysfunction [58, 69], VSMC contraction [89], VSMC proliferation and migration in the media [90], and accumulation of inflammatory cells in the adventitia [86]. Those Rho-kinase-mediated cellular responses lead to the development of vascular disease. In fact, mRNA expression of ROCKs is enhanced at the inflammatory and arteriosclerotic arterial lesions in animals [89] and humans [91]. In the context of atherosclerosis, Rho-kinase should be regarded as a pro-inflammatory and pro-atherogenic molecule. Thus, Rho-kinase is an important new therapeutic target for the treatment of atherosclerosis (Fig. 2.2).

2.7 Rho-Kinase in Myocardial Ischemia and Heart Failure

ROS production and Rho-kinase activation play a crucial role in myocardial damage after ischemia/reperfusion. Consistently, we have demonstrated that pretreatment with fasudil before reperfusion prevents endothelial dysfunction and reduces myocardial infarction size in dogs in vivo [92]. The beneficial effect of fasudil has also been demonstrated in a rabbit model of myocardial ischemia induced by intravenous administration of endothelin-1 [93], a canine model of pacing-induced myocardial ischemia [94], and a rat model of vasopressin-induced chronic myocardial ischemia [95]. AngII plays a key role in many physiological and pathological processes in cardiac cells, including cardiac hypertrophy [96]. Understanding the molecular mechanisms for AngII-induced myocardial disorders is important to develop new therapies for cardiac dysfunction [97]. One important mechanism now recognized to be involved in AngII-induced cardiac hypertrophy is ROS production [98, 99], however, the precise mechanism by which ROS cause myocardial hypertrophy and dysfunction still remains to be fully elucidated [100]. It has been demonstrated that cardiac troponin is a substrate of Rho-kinase [101]. Rho-kinase phosphorylates troponin and inhibits tension generation in cardiomyocytes. We have demonstrated that Rho-kinase inhibition with fasudil suppresses the development of cardiac hypertrophy and diastolic heart failure in Dahl salt-sensitive rats [102]. In patients with heart failure, intra-arterial infusion of fasudil caused preferential increase in forearm blood flow as compared with control subjects, suggesting an involvement of

Rho-kinase in the increased peripheral vascular resistance in patients with heart failure [103].

2.8 Rho-Kinase in Hypertension and Pulmonary Hypertension

Short-term administration of Y-27632, another Rho-kinase inhibitor, preferentially reduces systemic blood pressure in a dose-dependent manner in rat models of systemic hypertension, suggesting an involvement of Rho-kinase in the pathogenesis of hypertension [37]. The expression of Rho-kinase was significantly increased in spontaneously hypertensive rats (SHR) [104]. Local administration of a small amount of hydroxyfasudil into the nucleus tractus solitarii of the brain stem causes sustained decrease in heart rate and blood pressure in SHR but not in normotensive rats, suggesting that Rho-kinase is involved in the central mechanisms of sympathetic nerve activity [105]. Inhibition of Rho-kinase in the brain stem also augments baroreflex control of heart rate in rats [106]. Pulmonary hypertension (PH) is associated with hypoxic exposure, endothelial dysfunction, VSMC hypercontraction and proliferation, enhanced ROS production, and inflammatory cell migration, for which Rho-kinase may also be substantially involved. Indeed, long-term treatment with fasudil suppresses the development of monocrotaline-induced PH in rats [107] and of hypoxia-induced PH in mice [108]. Recently, we were able to obtain direct evidence for Rho-kinase activation in patients with pulmonary arterial hypertension (PAH) [109]. Furthermore, intravenous infusion of fasudil significantly reduced pulmonary vascular resistance in patients with PAH, indicating an involvement of Rho-kinase in the pathogenesis of PAH in humans [110].

2.9 Conclusions

Accumulating evidence has indicated that Rho-kinase plays important roles in the pathogenesis of a wide range of cardiovascular diseases in general and coronary vasomotion abnormalities in particular. Additionally, Rho-kinase inhibitors are useful for the treatment of those cardiovascular diseases. In conclusion, accumulating experimental and clinical evidence indicates that Rho-kinase is an important new target for the treatment of VSA and cardiovascular diseases.

Acknowledgements This work was supported in part by the grants-in-aid for Scientific Research (15H02535, 15H04816, and 15K15046), all of which are from the Ministry of Education, Culture, Sports, Science and Technology, Tokyo, Japan, the grants-in-aid for Scientific Research from the Ministry of Health, Labour, and Welfare, Tokyo, Japan (10102895), and the grants-in-aid for Scientific Research from the Japan Agency for Medical Research and Development, Tokyo, Japan (15ak0101035h0001, 16ek0109176h0001, 17ek0109227h0001).

References

1. Shimokawa H, Tomoike H, Nabeyama S, Yamamoto H, Araki H, Nakamura M, Ishii Y, Tanaka K. Coronary artery spasm induced in atherosclerotic miniature swine. Science. 1983;221(4610):560–2. https://doi.org/10.1126/science.6408736.
2. Shimokawa H, Ito A, Fukumoto Y, Kadokami T, Nakaike R, Sakata M, Takayanagi T, Egashira K, Takeshita A. Chronic treatment with interleukin-1β induces coronary intimal lesions and vasospastic responses in pigs in vivo. The role of platelet-derived growth factor. J Clin Invest. 1996;97(3):769–76. https://doi.org/10.1172/JCI118476.
3. Sato M, Tani E, Fujikawa H, Kaibuchi K. Involvement of Rho-kinase-mediated phosphorylation of myosin light chain in enhancement of cerebral vasospasm. Circ Res. 2000;87(3):195–200. https://www.ahajournals.org/doi/10.1161/01.RES.87.3.195.
4. Takagi Y, Yasuda S, Takahashi J, Takeda M, Nakayama M, Ito K, Hirose M, Wakayama Y, Fukuda K, Shimokawa H. Importance of dual induction tests for coronary vasospasm and ventricular fibrillation in patients surviving out-of-hospital cardiac arrest. Circ J. 2009;73(4):767–9. https://doi.org/10.1253/circj.CJ-09-0061.
5. Hizume T, Morikawa K, Takaki A, Abe K, Sunagawa K, Amano M, Kaibuchi K, Kubo C, Shimokawa H. Sustained elevation of serum cortisol level causes sensitization of coronary vasoconstricting responses in pigs in vivo: a possible link between stress and coronary vasospasm. Circ Res. 2006;99(7):767–75. https://doi.org/10.1161/01.RES.0000244093.69985.2f.
6. Kandabashi T, Shimokawa H, Miyata K, Kunihiro I, Kawano Y, Fukata Y, Higo T, Egashira K, Takahashi S, Kaibuchi K, Takeshita A. Inhibition of myosin phosphatase by upregulated Rho-kinase plays a key role for coronary artery spasm in a porcine model with interleukin-1β. Circulation. 2000;101(11):1319–23. https://doi.org/10.1161/01.CIR.101.11.1319.
7. Katsumata N, Shimokawa H, Seto M, Kozai T, Yamawaki T, Kuwata K, Egashira K, Ikegaki I, Asano T, Sasaki Y, Takeshita A. Enhanced myosin light chain phosphorylations as a central mechanism for coronary artery spasm in a swine model with interleukin-1β. Circulation. 1997;96(12):4357–63. https://doi.org/10.1161/01.cir.96.12.4357.
8. Shimokawa H, Seto M, Katsumata N, Amano M, Kozai T, Yamawaki T, Kuwata K, Kandabashi T, Egashira K, Ikegaki I, Asano T, Kaibuchi K, Takeshita A. Rho-kinase-mediated pathway induces enhanced myosin light chain phosphorylations in a swine model of coronary artery spasm. Cardiovasc Res. 1999;43(4):1029–39. https://doi.org/10.1016/s0008-6363(99)00144-3.
9. Masumoto A, Mohri M, Shimokawa H, Urakami L, Usui M, Takeshita A. Suppression of coronary artery spasm by the Rho-kinase inhibitor fasudil in patients with vasospastic angina. Circulation. 2002;105(13):1545–7. https://doi.org/10.1161/hc1002.105938.
10. Mohri M, Shimokawa H, Hirakawa Y, Masumoto A, Takeshita A. Rho-kinase inhibition with intracoronary fasudil prevents myocardial ischemia in patients with coronary microvascular spasm. J Am Coll Cardiol. 2003;41(1):15–9. https://doi.org/10.1016/S0735-1097(02)02632-3.
11. Shimokawa H, Hiramori K, Iinuma H, Hosoda S, Kishida H, Osada H, Katagiri T, Yamauchi K, Yui Y, Minamino T, Nakashima M, Kato K. Anti-anginal effect of fasudil, a Rho-kinase inhibitor, in patients with stable effort angina: a multicenter study. J Cardiovasc Pharmacol. 2002;40(5):751–61. https://doi.org/10.1097/00005344-200211000-00013.
12. Kikuchi Y, Yasuda S, Aizawa K, Tsuburaya R, Ito Y, Takeda M, Nakayama M, Ito K, Takahashi J, Shimokawa H. Enhanced Rho-kinase activity in circulating neutrophils of patients with vasospastic angina: a possible biomarker for diagnosis and disease activity assessment. J Am Coll Cardiol. 2011;58(12):1231–7. https://doi.org/10.1016/j.jacc.2011.05.046.
13. Fukata Y, Amano M, Kaibuchi K. Rho-Rho-kinase pathway in smooth muscle contraction and cytoskeletal reorganization of non-muscle cells. Trends Pharmacol Sci. 2001;22(1):32–9. https://doi.org/10.1016/s0165-6147(00)01596-0.
14. Takai Y, Sasaki T, Matozaki T. Small GTP-binding proteins. Physiol Rev. 2001;81(1):153–208. https://doi.org/10.1152/physrev.2001.81.1.153.

15. Loirand G, Pacaud P. The role of Rho protein signaling in hypertension. Nat Rev Cardiol. 2010;7(11):637–47. https://doi.org/10.1038/nrcardio.2010.136.
16. Etienne-Manneville S, Hall A. Rho GTPases in cell biology. Nature. 2002;420(6916):629–35. https://doi.org/10.1038/nature01148.
17. Schmidt A, Hall A. Guanine nucleotide exchange factors for Rho GTPases: turning on the switch. Genes Dev. 2002;16(13):1587–609. https://doi.org/10.1101/gad.1003302.
18. Bernards A. GAPs galore! A survey of putative Ras superfamily GTPase activating proteins in man and Drosophila. Biochim Biophys Acta. 2003;1603(2):47–82. https://doi.org/10.1016/s0304-419x(02)00082-3.
19. Olofsson B. Rho guanine dissociation inhibitors: pivotal molecules in cellular signalling. Cell Signal. 1999;11(8):545–54. https://doi.org/10.1016/s0898-6568(98)00063-1.
20. Kimura K, Ito M, Amano M, Chihara K, Fukata Y, Nakafuku M, Yamamori B, Feng J, Nakano T, Okawa K, Iwamatsu A, Kaibuchi K. Regulation of myosin phosphatase by Rho and Rho-associated kinase (Rho-kinase). Science. 1996;273(5272):245–8. https://doi.org/10.1126/science.273.5272.245.
21. Ishizaki T, Maekawa M, Fujisawa K, Okawa K, Iwamatsu A, Fujita A, Watanabe N, Saito Y, Kakizuka A, Morii N, Narumiya S. The small GTP-binding protein Rho binds to and activates a 160 kDa Ser/Thr protein kinase homologous to myotonic dystrophy kinase. EMBO J. 1996;15(8):1885–93.
22. Leung T, Chen XQ, Manser E, Lim L. The p160 RhoA-binding kinase ROKα is a member of a kinase family and is involved in the reorganization of the cytoskeleton. Mol Cell Biol. 1996;16(10):5313–27. https://doi.org/10.1128/mcb.16.10.5313.
23. Shimokawa H, Sunamura S, Satoh K. RhoA/Rho-kinase in the cardiovascular system. Circ Res. 2016;118(2):352–66. https://doi.org/10.1161/CIRCRESAHA.115.306532.
24. Kina-Tanada M, Sakanashi M, Tanimoto A, Kaname T, Matsuzaki T, Noguchi K, Uchida T, Nakasone J, Kozuka C, Ishida M, Kubota H, Taira Y, Totsuka Y, Kina SI, Sunakawa H, Omura J, Satoh K, Shimokawa H, Yanagihara N, Maeda S, Ohya Y, Matsushita M, Masuzaki H, Arasaki A, Tsutsui M. Long-term dietary nitrite and nitrate deficiency causes the metabolic syndrome, endothelial dysfunction and cardiovascular death in mice. Diabetologia. 2017;60(6):1138–51. https://doi.org/10.1007/s00125-017-4259-6.
25. Shimokawa H. Primary endothelial dysfunction: atherosclerosis. J Mol Cell Cardiol. 1999;31(1):23–37. https://doi.org/10.1006/jmcc.1998.0841.
26. Vanhoutte PM. Endothelium-derived free radicals: for worse and for better. J Clin Invest. 2001;107(1):23–5. https://doi.org/10.1172/JCI11832.
27. Shimokawa H. 2014 Williams Harvey lecture: importance of coronary vasomotion abnormalities -from bench to bedside. Eur Heart J. 2014;35(45):3180–93. https://doi.org/10.1093/eurheartj/ehu427.
28. Shimokawa H, Satoh K. Light and dark of reactive oxygen species for vascular function. J Cardiovasc Pharmacol. 2015;65(5):412–8. https://doi.org/10.1097/FJC.0000000000000159.
29. Shimokawa H, Satoh K. Vascular function. Arterioscler Thromb Vasc Biol. 2014;34(11):2359–62. https://doi.org/10.1161/ATVBAHA.114.304119.
30. Shimizu T, Fukumoto Y, Tanaka S, Satoh K, Ikeda S, Shimokawa H. Crucial role of ROCK2 in vascular smooth muscle cells for hypoxia-induced pulmonary hypertension in mice. Arterioscler Thromb Vasc Biol. 2013;33(12):2780–91. https://doi.org/10.1161/ATVBAHA.113.301357.
31. Do e Z, Fukumoto Y, Sugimura K, Miura Y, Tatebe S, Yamamoto S, Aoki T, Nochioka K, Nergui S, Yaoita N, Satoh K, Kondo M, Nakano M, Wakayama Y, Fukuda K, Nihei T, Kikuchi Y, Takahashi J, Shimokawa H. Rho-kinase activation in patients with heart failure. Circ J. 2013;77(10):2542–50. https://doi.org/10.1253/circj.CJ-13-0397.
32. Enkhjargal B, Godo S, Sawada A, Suvd N, Saito H, Noda K, Satoh K, Shimokawa H. Endothelial AMP-activated protein kinase regulates blood pressure and coronary flow responses through hyperpolarization mechanism in mice. Arterioscler Thromb Vasc Biol. 2014;34(7):1505–13. https://doi.org/10.1161/ATVBAHA.114.303735.

33. Shimokawa H, Takeshita A. Rho-kinase is an important therapeutic target in cardiovascular medicine. Arterioscler Thromb Vasc Biol. 2005;25(9):1767–75. https://doi.org/10.1161/01. ATV.0000176193.83629.c8.

34. Leung T, Manser E, Tan L, Lim L. A novel serine/threonine kinase binding the Ras-related RhoA GTPase which translocates the kinase to peripheral membranes. J Biol Chem. 1995;270(49):29051–4. https://doi.org/10.1074/jbc.270.49.29051.

35. Matsui T, Amano M, Yamamoto T, Chihara K, Nakafuku M, Ito M, Nakano T, Okawa K, Iwamatsu A, Kaibuchi K. Rho-associated kinase, a novel serine/threonine kinase, as a putative target for small GTP binding protein Rho. EMBO J. 1996;15(9):2208–16. https://doi.org/10.1002/j.1460-2075.1996.tb00574.x.

36. Nakagawa O, Fujisawa K, Ishizaki T, Saito Y, Nakao K, Narumiya S. ROCK-I and ROCK-II, two isoforms of Rho-associated coiled-coil forming protein serine/threonine kinase in mice. FEBS Lett. 1996;392(2):189–93. https://doi.org/10.1016/0014-5793(96)00811-3.

37. Uehata M, Ishizaki T, Satoh H, Ono T, Kawahara T, Morishita T, Tamakawa H, Yamagami K, Inui J, Maekawa M, Narumiya S. Calcium sensitization of smooth muscle mediated by a Rho-associated protein kinase in hypertension. Nature. 1997;389(6654):990–4. https://doi.org/10.1038/40187.

38. Davies SP, Reddy H, Caivano M, Cohen P. Specificity and mechanism of action of some commonly used protein kinase inhibitors. Biochem J. 2000;351(Pt 1):95–105. https://doi.org/10.1042/0264-6021:3510095.

39. Higashi M, Shimokawa H, Hattori T, Hiroki J, Mukai Y, Morikawa K, Ichiki T, Takahashi S, Takeshita A. Long-term inhibition of Rho-kinase suppresses angiotensin II-induced cardiovascular hypertrophy in rats in vivo: effect on endothelial NAD(P)H oxidase system. Circ Res. 2003;93(8):767–75. https://doi.org/10.1161/01.RES.0000096650.91688.28.

40. Coleman ML, Sahai EA, Yeo M, Bosch M, Dewar A, Olson MF. Membrane blebbing during apoptosis results from caspase-mediated activation of ROCK I. Nat Cell Biol. 2001;3(4):339–45. https://doi.org/10.1038/35070009.

41. Sebbagh M, Hamelin J, Bertoglio J, Solary E, Breard J. Direct cleavage of ROCK II by granzyme B induces target cell membrane blebbing in a caspase-independent manner. J Exp Med. 2005;201(3):465–71. https://doi.org/10.1084/jem.20031877.

42. Komander D, Garg R, Wan PT, Ridley AJ, Barford D. Mechanism of multi-site phosphorylation from a ROCK-I:RhoE complex structure. EMBO J. 2008;27(23):3175–85. https://doi.org/10.1038/emboj.2008.226.

43. Wang Y, Zheng XR, Riddick N, Bryden M, Baur W, Zhang X, Surks HK. ROCK isoform regulation of myosin phosphatase and contractility in vascular smooth muscle cells. Circ Res. 2009;104(4):531–40. https://doi.org/10.1161/CIRCRESAHA.108.188524.

44. Riento K, Guasch RM, Garg R, Jin B, Ridley AJ. RhoE binds to ROCK I and inhibits downstream signaling. Mol Cell Biol. 2003;23(12):4219–29. https://doi.org/10.1128/mcb.23.12.4219-4229.2003.

45. Hiroki J, Shimokawa H, Higashi M, Morikawa K, Kandabashi T, Kawamura N, Kubota T, Ichiki T, Amano M, Kaibuchi K, Takeshita A. Inflammatory stimuli upregulate Rho-kinase in human coronary vascular smooth muscle cells. J Mol Cell Cardiol. 2004;37(2):537–46. https://doi.org/10.1016/j.yjmcc.2004.05.008.

46. Loirand G, Guerin P, Pacaud P. Rho kinases in cardiovascular physiology and pathophysiology. Circ Res. 2006;98(3):322–34. https://doi.org/10.1161/01.RES.0000201960.04223.3c.

47. Riento K, Ridley AJ. ROCKs: multifunctional kinases in cell behaviour. Nat Rev Mol Cell Biol. 2003;4(6):446–56. https://doi.org/10.1038/nrm1128.

48. Thumkeo D, Keel J, Ishizaki T, Hirose M, Nonomura K, Oshima H, Oshima M, Taketo MM, Narumiya S. Targeted disruption of the mouse Rho-associated kinase 2 gene results in intrauterine growth retardation and fetal death. Mol Cell Biol. 2003;23(14):5043–55. https://doi.org/10.1128/mcb.23.14.5043-5055.2003.

49. Shimizu Y, Thumkeo D, Keel J, Ishizaki T, Oshima H, Oshima M, Noda Y, Matsumura F, Taketo MM, Narumiya S. ROCK-I regulates closure of the eyelids and ventral body wall

by inducing assembly of actomyosin bundles. J Cell Biol. 2005;168(6):941–53. https://doi. org/10.1083/jcb.200411179.

50. Liao JK, Seto M, Noma K. Rho kinase (ROCK) inhibitors. J Cardiovasc Pharmacol. 2007;50(1):17–24. https://doi.org/10.1097/FJC.0b013e318070d1bd.

51. Noma K, Rikitake Y, Oyama N, Yan G, Alcaide P, Liu PY, Wang H, Ahl D, Sawada N, Okamoto R, Hiroi Y, Shimizu K, Luscinskas FW, Sun J, Liao JK. ROCK1 mediates leukocyte recruitment and neointima formation following vascular injury. J Clin Invest. 2008;118(5):1632–44. https://doi.org/10.1172/JCI29226.

52. Zhou Q, Gensch C, Liao JK. Rho-associated coiled-coil-forming kinases (ROCKs): potential targets for the treatment of atherosclerosis and vascular disease. Trends Pharmacol Sci. 2011;32(3):167–73. https://doi.org/10.1016/j.tips.2010.12.006.

53. Radeff JM, Nagy Z, Stern PH. Rho and Rho kinase are involved in parathyroid hormone-stimulated protein kinase C α translocation and IL-6 promoter activity in osteoblastic cells. J Bone Miner Res. 2004;19(11):1882–91. https://doi.org/10.1359/jbmr.040806.

54. Funakoshi Y, Ichiki T, Shimokawa H, Egashira K, Takeda K, Kaibuchi K, Takeya M, Yoshimura T, Takeshita A. Rho-kinase mediates angiotensin II-induced monocyte chemoattractant protein-1 expression in rat vascular smooth muscle cells. Hypertension. 2001;38(1):100–4. https://doi.org/10.1161/01.hyp.38.1.100.

55. Hattori T, Shimokawa H, Higashi M, Hiroki J, Mukai Y, Kaibuchi K, Takeshita A. Long-term treatment with a specific Rho-kinase inhibitor suppresses cardiac allograft vasculopathy in mice. Circ Res. 2004;94(1):46–52. https://doi.org/10.1161/01.RES.0000107196.21335.2B.

56. Hattori T, Shimokawa H, Higashi M, Hiroki J, Mukai Y, Tsutsui H, Kaibuchi K, Takeshita A. Long-term inhibition of Rho-kinase suppresses left ventricular remodeling after myocardial infarction in mice. Circulation. 2004;109(18):2234–9. https://doi.org/10.1161/01. CIR.0000127939.16111.58.

57. Wang F, Okamoto Y, Inoki I, Yoshioka K, Du W, Qi X, Takuwa N, Gonda K, Yamamoto Y, Ohkawa R, Nishiuchi T, Sugimoto N, Yatomi Y, Mitsumori K, Asano M, Kinoshita M, Takuwa Y. Sphingosine-1-phosphate receptor-2 deficiency leads to inhibition of macrophage proinflammatory activities and atherosclerosis in apoE-deficient mice. J Clin Invest. 2010;120(11):3979–95. https://doi.org/10.1172/jci42315.

58. Takemoto M, Sun J, Hiroki J, Shimokawa H, Liao JK. Rho-kinase mediates hypoxia-induced downregulation of endothelial nitric oxide synthase. Circulation. 2002;106(1):57–62. https:// doi.org/10.1161/01.CIR.0000020682.73694.AB.

59. Oi K, Shimokawa H, Hiroki J, Uwatoku T, Abe K, Matsumoto Y, Nakajima Y, Nakajima K, Takeichi S, Takeshita A. Remnant lipoproteins from patients with sudden cardiac death enhance coronary vasospastic activity through upregulation of Rho-kinase. Arterioscler Thromb Vasc Biol. 2004;24(5):918–22. https://doi.org/10.1161/01.atv.0000126678.93747.80.

60. Mackay DJ, Hall A. Rho GTPases. J Biol Chem. 1998;273(33):20685–8. https://doi. org/10.1074/jbc.273.33.20685.

61. Neco P, Giner D, Viniegra S, Borges R, Villarroel A, Gutierrez LM. New roles of myosin II during vesicle transport and fusion in chromaffin cells. J Biol Chem. 2004;279(26):27450–7. https://doi.org/10.1074/jbc.M311462200.

62. Omar HA, Cherry PD, Mortelliti MP, Burke-Wolin T, Wolin MS. Inhibition of coronary artery superoxide dismutase attenuates endothelium-dependent and -independent nitrovasodilator relaxation. Circ Res. 1991;69(3):601–8. https://doi.org/10.1161/01.RES.69.3.601.

63. Alexander RW. Theodore Cooper memorial lecture. Hypertension and the pathogenesis of atherosclerosis. Oxidative stress and the mediation of arterial inflammatory response: a new perspective. Hypertension. 1995;25(2):155–61. https://doi.org/10.1161/01.hyp.25.2.155.

64. Baas AS, Berk BC. Differential activation of mitogen-activated protein kinases by H_2O_2 and O_2^- in vascular smooth muscle cells. Circ Res. 1995;77(1):29–36. https://doi.org/10.1161/01. res.77.1.29.

65. Griendling KK, Minieri CA, Ollerenshaw JD, Alexander RW. Angiotensin II stimulates NADH and NADPH oxidase activity in cultured vascular smooth muscle cells. Circ Res. 1994;74(6):1141–8. https://doi.org/10.1161/01.res.74.6.1141.

66. Takeda K, Ichiki T, Tokunou T, Iino N, Fujii S, Kitabatake A, Shimokawa H, Takeshita A. Critical role of Rho-kinase and MEK/ERK pathways for angiotensin II-induced plasminogen activator inhibitor type-1 gene expression. Arterioscler Thromb Vasc Biol. 2001;21(5):868–73. https://doi.org/10.1161/01.ATV.21.5.868.

67. Guilluy C, Bregeon J, Toumaniantz G, Rolli-Derkinderen M, Retailleau K, Loufrani L, Henrion D, Scalbert E, Bril A, Torres RM, Offermanns S, Pacaud P, Loirand G. The Rho exchange factor Arhgef1 mediates the effects of angiotensin II on vascular tone and blood pressure. Nat Med. 2010;16(2):183–90. https://doi.org/10.1038/nm.2079.

68. Seasholtz TM, Majumdar M, Kaplan DD, Brown JH. Rho and Rho kinase mediate thrombin-stimulated vascular smooth muscle cell DNA synthesis and migration. Circ Res. 1999;84(10):1186–93. https://doi.org/10.1161/01.RES.84.10.1186.

69. van Nieuw Amerongen GP, van Delft S, Vermeer MA, Collard JG, van Hinsbergh VW. Activation of RhoA by thrombin in endothelial hyperpermeability: role of Rho-kinase and protein tyrosine kinases. Circ Res. 2000;87(4):335–40. https://doi.org/10.1161/01.RES.87.4.335.

70. Kishi H, Bao J, Kohama K. Inhibitory effects of ML-9, wortmannin, and Y-27632 on the chemotaxis of vascular smooth muscle cells in response to platelet-derived growth factor-BB. J Biochem. 2000;128(5):719–22. https://doi.org/10.1093/oxfordjournals.jbchem.a022806.

71. Sauzeau V, Le Jeune H, Cario-Toumaniantz C, Vaillant N, Gadeau AP, Desgranges C, Scalbert E, Chardin P, Pacaud P, Loirand G. P2Y$_1$, P2Y$_2$, P2Y$_4$, and P2Y$_6$ receptors are coupled to Rho and Rho kinase activation in vascular myocytes. Am J Physiol Heart Circ Physiol. 2000;278(6):H1751–61. https://doi.org/10.1152/ajpheart.2000.278.6.H1751.

72. Sauzeau V, Le Mellionnec E, Bertoglio J, Scalbert E, Pacaud P, Loirand G. Human urotensin II-induced contraction and arterial smooth muscle cell proliferation are mediated by RhoA and Rho-kinase. Circ Res. 2001;88(11):1102–4. https://doi.org/10.1161/hh1101.092034.

73. Takemoto M, Liao JK. Pleiotropic effects of 3-hydroxy-3-methylglutaryl coenzyme a reductase inhibitors. Arterioscler Thromb Vasc Biol. 2001;21(11):1712–9. https://doi.org/10.1161/hq1101.098486.

74. Shimokawa H. Cellular and molecular mechanisms of coronary artery spasm: lessons from animal models. Jpn Circ J. 2000;64(1):1–12. https://doi.org/10.1007/978-3-642-56225-9_56.

75. Shimokawa H. Rho-kinase as a novel therapeutic target in treatment of cardiovascular diseases. J Cardiovasc Pharmacol. 2002;39(3):319–27. https://doi.org/10.1097/00005344-200203000-00001.

76. Amano M, Chihara K, Kimura K, Fukata Y, Nakamura N, Matsuura Y, Kaibuchi K. Formation of actin stress fibers and focal adhesions enhanced by Rho-kinase. Science. 1997;275(5304):1308–11. https://doi.org/10.1126/science.275.5304.1308.

77. Hall A. Rho GTPases and the actin cytoskeleton. Science. 1998;279(5350):509–14. https://doi.org/10.1126/science.279.5350.509.

78. Rao GN, Berk BC. Active oxygen species stimulate vascular smooth muscle cell growth and proto-oncogene expression. Circ Res. 1992;70(3):593–9. https://doi.org/10.1161/01.res.70.3.593.

79. Ross R. Atherosclerosis is an inflammatory disease. Am Heart J. 1999;138(5 Pt 2):S419–20. https://doi.org/10.1016/s0002-8703(99)70266-8.

80. Libby P. Inflammation in atherosclerosis. Nature. 2002;420(6917):868–74. https://doi.org/10.1038/nature01323.

81. Inoue T, Node K. Molecular basis of restenosis and novel issues of drug-eluting stents. Circ J. 2009;73(4):615–21. https://doi.org/10.1253/circj.cj-09-0059.

82. Shimokawa H, Rashid M. Development of Rho-kinase inhibitors for cardiovascular medicine. Trends Pharmacol Sci. 2007;28(6):296–302. https://doi.org/10.1016/j.tips.2007.04.006.

83. Eto Y, Shimokawa H, Hiroki J, Morishige K, Kandabashi T, Matsumoto Y, Amano M, Hoshijima M, Kaibuchi K, Takeshita A. Gene transfer of dominant negative Rho-kinase suppresses neointimal formation after balloon injury in pigs. Am J Physiol Heart Circ Physiol. 2000;278(6):H1744–50. https://doi.org/10.1152/ajpheart.2000.278.6.H1744.

84. Sawada N, Itoh H, Ueyama K, Yamashita J, Doi K, Chun TH, Inoue M, Masatsugu K, Saito T, Fukunaga Y, Sakaguchi S, Arai H, Ohno N, Komeda M, Nakao K. Inhibition of Rho-associated kinase results in suppression of neointimal formation of balloon-injured arteries. Circulation. 2000;101(17):2030–3. https://doi.org/10.1161/01.cir.101.17.2030.

85. Shibata R, Kai H, Seki Y, Kato S, Morimatsu M, Kaibuchi K, Imaizumi T. Role of Rho-associated kinase in neointima formation after vascular injury. Circulation. 2001;103(2):284–9. https://doi.org/10.1161/01.CIR.103.2.284.

86. Miyata K, Shimokawa H, Kandabashi T, Higo T, Morishige K, Eto Y, Egashira K, Kaibuchi K, Takeshita A. Rho-kinase is involved in macrophage-mediated formation of coronary vascular lesions in pigs in vivo. Arterioscler Thromb Vasc Biol. 2000;20(11):2351–8. https://doi.org/10.1161/01.atv.20.11.2351.

87. Shimokawa H, Morishige K, Miyata K, Kandabashi T, Eto Y, Ikegaki I, Asano T, Kaibuchi K, Takeshita A. Long-term inhibition of Rho-kinase induces a regression of arteriosclerotic coronary lesions in a porcine model in vivo. Cardiovasc Res. 2001;51(1):169–77. https://doi.org/10.1016/S0008-6363(01)00291-7.

88. Matsumoto Y, Uwatoku T, Oi K, Abe K, Hattori T, Morishige K, Eto Y, Fukumoto Y, Nakamura K, Shibata Y, Matsuda T, Takeshita A, Shimokawa H. Long-term inhibition of Rho-kinase suppresses neointimal formation after stent implantation in porcine coronary arteries: involvement of multiple mechanisms. Arterioscler Thromb Vasc Biol. 2004;24(1):181–6. https://doi.org/10.1161/01.atv.0000105053.46994.5b.

89. Kandabashi T, Shimokawa H, Miyata K, Kunihiro I, Eto Y, Morishige K, Matsumoto Y, Obara K, Nakayama K, Takahashi S, Takeshita A. Evidence for protein kinase C-mediated activation of Rho-kinase in a porcine model of coronary artery spasm. Arterioscler Thromb Vasc Biol. 2003;23(12):2209–14. https://doi.org/10.1161/01.ATV.0000104010.87348.26.

90. Yamakawa T, Tanaka S, Numaguchi K, Yamakawa Y, Motley ED, Ichihara S, Inagami T. Involvement of Rho-kinase in angiotensin II-induced hypertrophy of rat vascular smooth muscle cells. Hypertension. 2000;35(1 Pt 2):313–8. https://doi.org/10.1161/01.HYP.35.1.313.

91. Kandabashi T, Shimokawa H, Mukai Y, Matoba T, Kunihiro I, Morikawa K, Ito M, Takahashi S, Kaibuchi K, Takeshita A. Involvement of Rho-kinase in agonists-induced contractions of arteriosclerotic human arteries. Arterioscler Thromb Vasc Biol. 2002;22(2):243–8. https://doi.org/10.1161/hq0202.104274.

92. Yada T, Shimokawa H, Hiramatsu O, Kajita T, Shigeto F, Tanaka E, Shinozaki Y, Mori H, Kiyooka T, Katsura M, Ohkuma S, Goto M, Ogasawara Y, Kajiya F. Beneficial effect of hydroxyfasudil, a specific Rho-kinase inhibitor, on ischemia/reperfusion injury in canine coronary microcirculation in vivo. J Am Coll Cardiol. 2005;45(4):599–607. https://doi.org/10.1016/j.jacc.2004.10.053.

93. Sato S, Ikegaki I, Asano T, Shimokawa H. Antiischemic properties of fasudil in experimental models of vasospastic angina. Jpn J Pharmacol. 2001;87(1):34–40. https://doi.org/10.1254/jjp.87.34.

94. Utsunomiya T, Satoh S, Ikegaki I, Toshima Y, Asano T, Shimokawa H. Antianginal effects of hydroxyfasudil, a Rho-kinase inhibitor, in a canine model of effort angina. Br J Pharmacol. 2001;134(8):1724–30. https://doi.org/10.1038/sj.bjp.0704410.

95. Satoh S, Ikegaki I, Toshima Y, Watanabe A, Asano T, Shimokawa H. Effects of Rho-kinase inhibitor on vasopressin-induced chronic myocardial damage in rats. Life Sci. 2002;72(1):103–12. https://doi.org/10.1016/s0024-3205(02)02178-1.

96. Mehta PK, Griendling KK. Angiotensin II cell signaling: physiological and pathological effects in the cardiovascular system. Am J Physiol Cell Physiol. 2007;292(1):C82–97. https://doi.org/10.1152/ajpcell.00287.2006.

97. Sadoshima J, Xu Y, Slayter HS, Izumo S. Autocrine release of angiotensin II mediates stretch-induced hypertrophy of cardiac myocytes in vitro. Cell. 1993;75(5):977–84. https://doi.org/10.1016/0092-8674(93)90541-w.

98. Nakamura K, Fushimi K, Kouchi H, Mihara K, Miyazaki M, Ohe T, Namba M. Inhibitory effects of antioxidants on neonatal rat cardiac myocyte hypertrophy induced by tumor necrosis factor-α and angiotensin II. Circulation. 1998;98(8):794–9. https://doi.org/10.1161/01.CIR.98.8.794.

99. Akki A, Zhang M, Murdoch C, Brewer A, Shah AM. NADPH oxidase signaling and cardiac myocyte function. J Mol Cell Cardiol. 2009;47(1):15–22. https://doi.org/10.1016/j.yjmcc.2009.04.004.

100. Shibata R, Ouchi N, Murohara T. Adiponectin and cardiovascular disease. Circ J. 2009;73(4):608–14. https://doi.org/10.1253/circj.CJ-09-0057.

101. Vahebi S, Kobayashi T, Warren CM, de Tombe PP, Solaro RJ. Functional effects of Rho-kinase-dependent phosphorylation of specific sites on cardiac troponin. Circ Res. 2005;96(7):740–7. https://doi.org/10.1161/01.RES.0000162457.56568.7d.

102. Fukui S, Fukumoto Y, Suzuki J, Saji K, Nawata J, Tawara S, Shinozaki T, Kagaya Y, Shimokawa H. Long-term inhibition of Rho-kinase ameliorates diastolic heart failure in hypertensive rats. J Cardiovasc Pharmacol. 2008;51(3):317–26. https://doi.org/10.1097/FJC.0b013e31816533b7.

103. Kishi T, Hirooka Y, Masumoto A, Ito K, Kimura Y, Inokuchi K, Tagawa T, Shimokawa H, Takeshita A, Sunagawa K. Rho-kinase inhibitor improves increased vascular resistance and impaired vasodilation of the forearm in patients with heart failure. Circulation. 2005;111(21):2741–7. https://doi.org/10.1161/CIRCULATIONAHA.104.510248.

104. Mukai Y, Shimokawa H, Matoba T, Kandabashi T, Satoh S, Hiroki J, Kaibuchi K, Takeshita A. Involvement of Rho-kinase in hypertensive vascular disease: a novel therapeutic target in hypertension. FASEB J. 2001;15(6):1062–4. https://doi.org/10.1096/fsb2fj000735fje.

105. Ito K, Hirooka Y, Sakai K, Kishi T, Kaibuchi K, Shimokawa H, Takeshita A. Rho/Rho-kinase pathway in brain stem contributes to blood pressure regulation via sympathetic nervous system: possible involvement in neural mechanisms of hypertension. Circ Res. 2003;92(12):1337–43. https://doi.org/10.1161/01.RES.0000079941.59846.D4.

106. Ito K, Hirooka Y, Kishi T, Kimura Y, Kaibuchi K, Shimokawa H, Takeshita A. Rho/Rho-kinase pathway in the brainstem contributes to hypertension caused by chronic nitric oxide synthase inhibition. Hypertension. 2004;43(2):156–62. https://doi.org/10.1161/01.HYP.0000114602.82140.a4.

107. Abe K, Shimokawa H, Morikawa K, Uwatoku T, Oi K, Matsumoto Y, Hattori T, Nakashima Y, Kaibuchi K, Sueishi K, Takeshit A. Long-term treatment with a Rho-kinase inhibitor improves monocrotaline-induced fatal pulmonary hypertension in rats. Circ Res. 2004;94(3):385–93. https://doi.org/10.1161/01.RES.0000111804.34509.94.

108. Abe K, Tawara S, Oi K, Hizume T, Uwatoku T, Fukumoto Y, Kaibuchi K, Shimokawa H. Long-term inhibition of Rho-kinase ameliorates hypoxia-induced pulmonary hypertension in mice. J Cardiovasc Pharmacol. 2006;48(6):280–5. https://doi.org/10.1097/01.fjc.0000248244.64430.4a.

109. Do e Z, Fukumoto Y, Takaki A, Tawara S, Ohashi J, Nakano M, Tada T, Saji K, Sugimura K, Fujita H, Hoshikawa Y, Nawata J, Kondo T, Shimokawa H. Evidence for Rho-kinase activation in patients with pulmonary arterial hypertension. Circ J. 2009;73(9):1731–9. https://doi.org/10.1253/circj.cj-09-01350.

110. Fukumoto Y, Matoba T, Ito A, Tanaka H, Kishi T, Hayashidani S, Abe K, Takeshita A, Shimokawa H. Acute vasodilator effects of a Rho-kinase inhibitor, fasudil, in patients with severe pulmonary hypertension. Heart. 2005;91(3):391–2. https://doi.org/10.1007/s00380-009-1176-8.

Chapter 3
Diagnosis of Coronary Artery Spasm

**Kensuke Nishimiya, Yasuharu Matsumoto, Jun Takahashi,
and Hiroaki Shimokawa**

Abstract Seminal clinical studies have shown that percutaneous coronary inter-vention (PCI) in patients with stable angina gives few benefits as compared with optimal medical therapy alone (Boden et al., N Engl J Med 356:1503–1516, 2007; Al-Lamee et al., Lancet 391:31–40, 2018). Therefore, making diagnosis of coro-nary vasomotion abnormalities regardless of obstructive or nonobstructive arterial segments has dramatically increased its clinical significance. Coronary artery spasm plays a key role in a wide range of ischemic heart diseases not only in vasospastic angina (VSA) but also in acute coronary syndrome and sudden cardiac death. It is of importance to have the precise diagnostic criteria for coronary artery spasm based on the clinically available evaluation methods. Particularly, recent studies have made substantial contributions to the development of new approaches that can pre-dict the risk of future cardiovascular events in patients with VSA. Ample clinical evidence has been accumulated for elucidating the detailed mechanisms of coronary artery spasm in vivo. In this chapter, we will summarize recent advances in diagnos-tic methodology of coronary artery spasm.

Keywords Acetylcholine · Adventitia · Coronary artery spasm · the Coronary Artery Vasomotion Disorders International Study Group (COVAIDS) · Coronary microvascular dysfunction (CMD) · Ergonovine · 18F-fluorodeoxyglucose-positron emission tomography (FDG-PET) · the Japanese Coronary Spasm Association (JCSA) · Lactic acid · Optical coherence tomography (OCT) · Perivascular adipose tissue (PVAT) · Rho-kinase · Serotonin · Spasm provocation test · Vasa vasorum · Vasospastic angina (VSA).

K. Nishimiya · Y. Matsumoto · J. Takahashi · H. Shimokawa (✉)
Department of Cardiovascular Medicine, Tohoku University Graduate School of Medicine, Sendai, Miyagi, Japan
e-mail: shimo@cardio.med.tohoku.ac.jp

3.1 Clinical Definition and Diagnostic Criteria of Coronary Artery Spasm

Referring to the Japanese Circulation Society (JCS) guidelines for diagnosis and treatment of patients with VSA [1], definite VSA is diagnosed when ischemic changes on electrocardiogram (ECG), defined as a transient ST elevation of >0.1 mV, an ST depression of >0.1 mV, or new appearance of negative U waves in at least 2 contiguous leads, are documented during spontaneous angina attack. In case that ECG shows borderline ischemic change, definite VSA is angiographically diagnosed when transient, total, subtotal (>90% stenosis) of a coronary artery accompanied by angina pain and ischemic ECG change during the spasm provocation test with acetylcholine, ergonovine, or hyperventilation (Fig. 3.1). Following the JCS guidelines, a position paper from the Coronary Artery Vasomotion Disorders

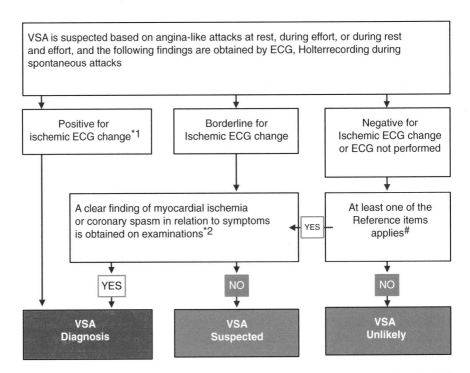

Fig. 3.1 Diagnosis of coronary artery spasm. Diagnostic algorithm of VSA (quoted from the JCS guidelines). *1Ischemic change is defined as a transient ST elevation of 0.1 mV or more, an ST depression of 0.1 mV or more, or new appearance of negative U waves, recorded in at least two contiguous leads on 12-lead ECG. *2Examinations include the drug-induced spasm provocation test during cardiac catheterization and hyperventilation test. A positive finding for coronary artery spasm on angiography in coronary artery spasm provocation test is defined as "transient, total, or subtotal occlusion (>90% stenosis) of a coronary artery with signs/symptoms of myocardial ischemia (anginal pain and ischemic ECG change)". *VSA* vasospastic angina, *ECG* electrocardiogram. (Reproduced from JCS joint working group [1])

International Study Group (COVAIDS) depicts regarding the physical assessment of VSA that (1) subjective symptoms often appear at rest, especially between night and early morning, (2) exercise tolerance is markedly reduced in morning, (3) hyperventilation relates to the symptoms, and (4) calcium-channel blockers suppress the symptoms [2].

3.2   Noninvasive Evaluation Methods

ECG and Holter ECG are useful for documentation of ECG changes regardless of the presence or the absence of symptoms (Class I) [1]. The criteria for positive ECG findings include ST-segment elevation/suppression of 0.1 mV or more in at least 2 contiguous leads on 12-lead ECG. Exercise or hyperventilation test, often recommended to perform in resting condition desirably in the morning, could be an option for noninvasive assessment for coronary artery spasm. Usefulness of noninvasive cardiovascular imaging tools, such as myocardial scintigraphy and multi detector-row computed tomography (CT), remains to be determined in future guidelines.

3.3   Pharmacological Spasm Provocative Tests

The JCS guidelines highly recommend spasm provocation tests with acetylcholine (Class I) when a patient is negative for noninvasive VSA evaluation but is still suspected for coronary artery spasm clinically [1]. In 1986, Yasue et al. reported the usefulness of pharmacological spasm provocation test with intracoronary acetylcholine to induce coronary spasm [3]. Notably, a high diagnostic accuracy of acetylcholine provocation test for patients with variant angina (sensitivity, 90%; specificity, 99%) was reported [4]. Recent papers from the Europe demonstrated that pharmacological spasm provocation tests with acetylcholine are safe and useful for making VSA diagnosis in white patients [5, 6]. Prior to the introduction of acetylcholine, intravenous ergonovine was originally reported in 1949 [7], and was used for the first spasm provocation testing in 1972 [8]. Ergonovine provocation test is recommended if patients have a contraindication to acetylcholine due to comorbid bronchial asthma or severe atrioventricular conduction disorder [9].

In 2006, the Japanese Coronary Spasm Association (JCSA) was established, in which 85 Japanese institutes participated and registered VSA patients between September 1, 2007 and December 31, 2008 [10]. Since then, the JCSA registry has provided robust evidence, especially in the clinical presentation of coronary artery spasm. First, a study by Takagi et al. reported the safety of the spasm provocation tests and found the significant correlation between angiographic findings and long-term prognosis in 1244 VSA patients who were diagnosed with pharmacological provocation tests with either intracoronary acetylcholine or ergonovine [11]. In this study, overall incidence of arrhythmic complications, such as ventricular tachycardia (VT) or ventricular fibrillation (VF) during the provocation tests, was 6.8%, which was comparable with those who were documented spontaneous angina attack. Patients who underwent acetylcholine provocation test showed a significant higher rate of arrhythmic complications as compared with those with ergonovine provocation test (acetylcholine 9.3% vs. ergonovine 3.2%, $P < 0.001$), which was more prominent for VT/VF (acetylcholine 4.9% vs. ergonovine 0.8%, $P < 0.001$). VSA patients with induced VT/VF during provocation test were characterized by a higher dose of acetylcholine use during the test, female, diffuse spasm in the right coronary artery, multivessel spasm, and lower prevalence of organic stenosis. When applied the logistic regression analysis, acetylcholine use during the provocation tests and diffuse spasm in the right coronary artery were strong correlated factors for the occurrence of provocation-related VT/VF. In contrast, the 5-year survival rate free from major adverse cardiac events (MACEs), including cardiac death, non-fatal myocardial infarction, hospitalization due to unstable angina pectoris and heart failure, and appropriate implantable cardioverter-defibrillator (ICD) shocks during the follow-up period, was 92%, and that of all-cause death was 98%. Importantly, MACE-free survival rate was statistically comparable between VSA patients with provocation-related VT/VF and those without them (Fig. 3.2). The multivariable Cox proportional hazard analysis showed that a mixture of focal and diffuse spasm observed in multivessels and organic stenosis were strongly correlated with MACEs, whereas no correlation between provocation-related arrhythmias and MACEs during the follow-up period was noted (Table 3.1). Thus, the JCSA study demonstrates an acceptable level of safety of the pharmacological spasm provocation test and its usefulness for the risk stratification of VSA patients [11].

Another landmark study form the JCSA registry developed the JCSA risk score that can provide comprehensive risk assessment and prognostic stratification for VSA patients [12]. A total of 7 variables, history of out-of-hospital cardiac arrest (4 points), smoking, rest angina alone, organic coronary stenosis, multivessel spasm during the spasm provocation tests (2 points each), ST-segment elevation during angina, and β-blocker use (1 point each) were chosen for the JCSA score. Intriguingly, MACE were incrementally documented in line with the low-risk, intermediate-risk, and high-risk (2.5%, 7.0%, and 13.0%, $P < 0.001$) (Fig. 3.3a). Among the 3 risk groups, clear prognostic utility of the JCSA scoring system for MACE was confirmed throughout the follow-up period (Fig. 3.3b). The study has thoroughly increased the importance of the spasm provocation test for the risk stratification of future cardiovascular events in VSA patients [12].

Although it has been believed for long time that VSA is more common in Asian countries compared with Western countries, recent studies from Germany revealed that the prevalence of VSA in Caucasians may be higher than previously thought [5, 6]. Heretofore, studies have suggested ethnic differences in the clinical manifestation and long-term prognosis of VSA patients between Japanese and Caucasians [13]. The JCSA study group recently revisited the ethnic differences in the VSA patient prognosis by comparing 1339 Japanese and 118 Caucasians [14]. The study performed by Sato et al. reported that spasm provocation tests were comparably performed in 95% of Japanese vs. 84% of Caucasians. Multivessel spasm was more

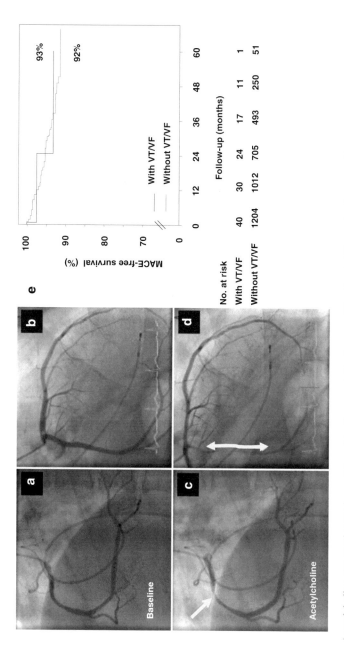

Fig. 3.2 Acetylcholine provocation testing and its safety. Representative images of focal and diffuse mixed type, multivessel spasm (**a–d**). Baseline angiography showing no significant organic stenosis in the right and left coronary arteries (**a**, **b**). Angiography after intracoronary administration of acetylcholine demonstrating focal spasm in the proximal segment of the right coronary artery (yellow allow in **c**) and diffuse spasm along the proximal and middle segments of the left circumflex coronary artery (yellow allow in **d**). The focal spasm is defined as a discrete luminal narrowing localized in the major coronary artery. The diffuse spasm was diagnosed when luminal narrowing was observed continuously from the proximal to the distal segment of the coronary artery. The mixed type is defined as the multivessel spasm in which at least one coronary artery had focal spasm and the other had diffuse spasm. The Kaplan–Meier curve for MACE and survival in VSA patients after the diagnosis with the provocation testing (**e**). MACE-free survival rate was comparable between patients with ventricular tachycardia (VT)/ventricular fibrillation (VF) (red line, $N = 40$) and those without it (blue line, $N = 1204$) ($P = 0.90$) (**e**). MACE includes cardiac death, nonfatal myocardial infarction, hospitalization due to unstable angina pectoris and heart failure, and appropriate implantable cardioverter-defibrillator (ICD) shocks during the follow-up period. (Reproduced from Takagi et al. [11])

Table 3.1 Factors correlated with major adverse cardiac events

	Multivariable analysis HR	95% CI	*P*-value
LAD spasm	1.22	0.72–2.05	0.46
LCX spasm	0.95	0.55–1.64	0.85
RCA spasm	1.25	0.75–2.08	0.40
Multivessel spasm	1.47	0.89–2.41	0.13
Type of spasm			
Focal single vessel	1.00	0.45–1.74	
Diffuse single vessel	0.88	0.04–1.74	0.72
Focal multivessel	0.27	0.04–1.99	0.20
Diffuse multivessel	1.15	0.58–2.31	0.69
Mixed multivessel	2.84	1.34–6.03	**0.006**
Organic stenosis			
Without stenosis	1.00		
Nonorganic stenosis	1.75	1.01–3.04	**0.048**
Significant stenosis	2.27	1.23–4.20	**0.009**
Provocation-related VT/VF	0.84	0.20–3.43	0.84
Provocation-related bradyarrhythmia	0.00	0.00–8.22	0.96

Variables were individually adjusted for age, sex, smoking, previous history of myocardial infarction, and history of out-of-hospital cardiac arrest. *LAD* left anterior descending, *LCX* left circumflex, *RCA* right coronary artery, *VT* ventricular tachycardia, *VF* ventricular fibrillation. (Reproduced from Takagi et al. [11])

prevalent in Japanese, whereas provocation-related arrhythmias were more common in Caucasians. The survival rate free from MACE, as described above, was significantly lower in Caucasians as compared with Japanese. In the multivariable analysis, the JCSA risk score, including the number of vessels positive for spasm provocation tests, was found to show good correlations with MACE rates in both Japanese and Caucasian patients, indicating the clinical importance of spasm provocation tests not only in Japan but also in Western countries.

In the context of the widespread utilization of drug-eluting stents (DES) in coronary intervention, it is fundamentally important to perform spasm provocation tests for patients with unremitting angina symptoms even after resolving the organic stenosis with DES implantation. An experimental study by Shiroto et al. demonstrated that a first-generation DES is likely to induce coronary hyperconstricting responses in response to intracoronary serotonin at the segments of proximal and distal edge of DES as compared with its platform bare-metal stents (BMS) in pigs in vivo, for which activated Rho-kinase plays an important role [15]. This finding was subsequently confirmed by a clinical study by Aizawa et al., demonstrating that pretreatment with fasudil, a selective Rho-kinase inhibitor, markedly inhibits acetylcholine-induced coronary hyperconstricting responses in patients implanted with DES in vivo [16]. More recently, a multicenter randomized control study by Tsuburaya et al. revealed that even everolimus-eluting stents, most widely used DES, could also induce coronary hyperconstricting responses at 8–10 months after implantation [17] (Fig. 3.4a, c). Intriguingly, long-term oral administration of

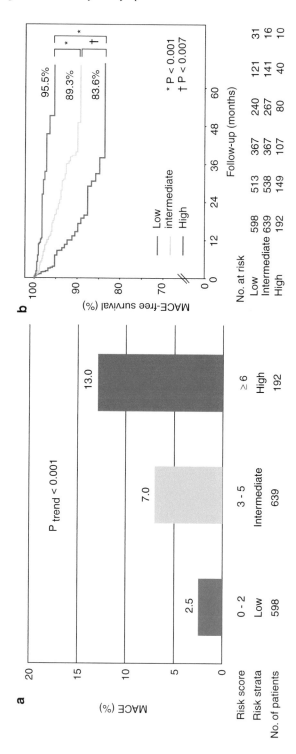

Fig. 3.3 The Japanese Coronary Spasm Association (JCSA) risk score. In the JCSA registry, VSA patients were classified into the 3 risk groups in accordance with the risk scoring system composed of history of out-of-hospital cardiac arrest (4 points), smoking, rest angina alone, organic coronary stenosis, and multi-vessel spasm during the spasm provocation tests (2 points per each), ST-segment elevation during angina and β-blocker use (1 point per each). The graph (**a**) showing the incidence of MACE as described in Fig. 3.2. The Kaplan–Meier curve for MACE among the 3 risk groups showing clear prognostic utility of the scoring system throughout the follow-up period (**b**). (Reproduced from Takagi et al. [12])

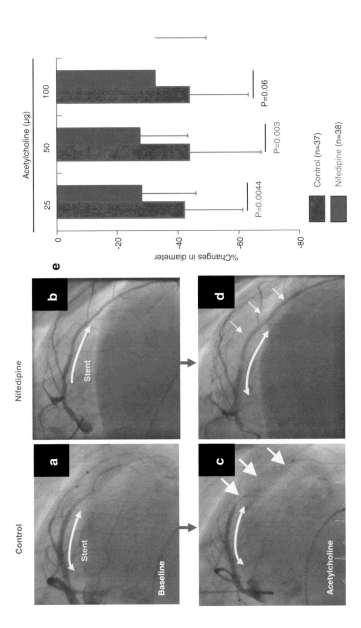

Fig. 3.4 Inhibitory effects of long-acting nifedipine on coronary hyperconstricting responses after everolimus-eluting stents implantation in patients with stable angina pectoris. Representative angiography of patients with an implanted everolimus-eluting stent for 8 months at the timing of baseline (**a**, **b**) and that after intracoronary administration of acetylcholine (**c**, **d**). Baseline angiography showing no significant in-stent restenosis in the left coronary arteries in both control and nifedipine-treated patients (**a**, **b**). Coronary hyperconstricting responses to acetylcholine were noted in the control patient (as indicated by yellow arrows in **c**), whereas such responses were suppressed in the patient of the nifedipine group (**d**). The results of quantitative coronary angiography for % changes in diameter of the segments distal to the stents before and after intracoronary acetylcholine (**e**), showing that coronary vasoconstricting responses to acetylcholine were significantly suppressed in the nifedipine group compared with the control group. (Reproduced from Tsuburaya et al. [17])

nifedipine, a long-acting calcium channel blocker, inhibited DES-induced coronary hyperconstricting responses (Fig. 3.4b, d, e). Nishimiya et al. also reported that improved biocompatibility of polymer coating may ameliorate such coronary vasomotion abnormalities after DES [18]. Given the high rate of patients (~40%) who suffer from chest pain even after coronary intervention, spasm provocation tests are strongly recommended for those with unremitting angina especially after DES implantation [19].

3.4   Biomarkers for Coronary Artery Spasm

Although the JCS guidelines state that it is useful for VSA and microvascular spasm diagnosis to detect inversion of lactic acid production by measuring lactate levels at a coronary artery vs. coronary sinus (Class IIIb) [1, 20], the measurement has been hampered by its inconvenience due to the requirement of catheter insertion into the coronary sinus. Thus, we also aimed to develop novel biomarkers for coronary artery spasm that can be easily used in the clinical setting. In order to clarify the existence of genetic linkage in the pathogenesis of coronary artery spasm, the frequencies of human leukocyte antigen (HLA) were examined in 37 patients with variant angina and 236 healthy controls, and were found to show no significant differences between the patients and the controls [21]. Hizume et al. reported that sustained elevation of serum cortisol level sensitizes coronary smooth muscle to serotonin to cause coronary vasospastic responses in pigs in vivo, suggesting the cross-link between stress and coronary artery spasm [22].

We were able to demonstrate that Rho-kinase activity in circulating neutrophils, determined by the extent of phosphorylation of myosin-binding subunit (MBS, a substrate of Rho-kinase), is significantly enhanced in VSA patients as compared with controls, which is a useful noninvasive diagnostic biomarker to assess the vasospastic activity [23] (Fig. 3.5a). In this study, Rho-kinase activity in circulating neutrophils was expressed as the ratio of phosphorylated MBS (p-MBS) to total MBS (t-MBS) (Fig. 3.5a, b). A p-MBS ratio of 1.18 was identified as the best cutoff level to predict the diagnosis of VSA (Fig. 3.5b). We also demonstrated that the Rho-kinase activity is able to show the severity of angina symptoms, and the responsiveness to medical treatment [23]. We also subsequently demonstrated that Rho-kinase activity in circulating neutrophils in VSA patients was temporally enhanced after the Great East Japan Earthquake associated with disaster-related mental stress (Fig. 3.5c) [24] and that the Rho-kinase activity well corresponds to distinct circadian variation in VSA patients (Fig. 3.5d) [25]. Moreover, when VSA patients were divided by a median value of Rho-kinase activity, VSA patients with higher Rho-kinase activity ($\geq$1.20) had significantly worse prognosis (Fig. 3.6a) [26]. In this study, a p-MBS ratio of 1.24 was identified as the best cutoff level to predict future cardiac events in VSA patients (Fig. 3.6b). Of note, combination of Rho-kinase activity with the JCSA risk score dramatically enhanced the prognostic impact in VSA patients [26].

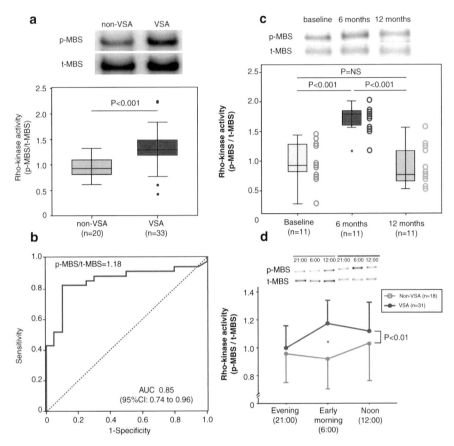

Fig. 3.5 Rho-kinase activity in circulating leukocytes of VSA patients (diagnosis). Rho-kinase activity in circulating neutrophils is determined by the extent of phosphorylation of myosin-binding subunit (MBS, a substrate of Rho-kinase), and is expressed as the ratio of phosphorylated MBS (p-MBS) to total MBS (t-MBS) (**a**, **b**). Rho-kinase activity was significantly enhanced in VSA patients compared with controls (**a**). Receiver-operating characteristic (ROC) curve analysis confirmed that a p-MBS ratio of 1.18 was identified as the best cutoff level to predict the diagnosis of VSA (**b**). (Reprinted with permission from Kikuchi et al. [23]). Changes in Rho-kinase activity in circulating neutrophils of VSA patients after the Great East Japan Earthquake (**c**). Rho-kinase activity was significantly increased at 6 months after the Earthquake and was returned to the baseline level at 12 months. Rho-kinase activity in circulating neutrophils well corresponded to circadian variation of disease activity in VSA patients (**d**). (Reproduced from Nihei et al. [24, 25])

Coronary microvascular dysfunction (CMD) has been emerging as an aggravating factor of cardiovascular disease [27, 28]. When no flow-limiting stenosis is noted on coronary angiography, coronary microcirculation can be assessed by index of microvascular resistance (IMR) [29]. We have recently demonstrated that comorbid CMD determined by increased IMR >18 worsens the long-term prognosis of VSA patients [30] (see Chap. 8 for details). In the study by Odaka et al., we obtained blood samples from the left coronary ostia before spasm provocation tests,

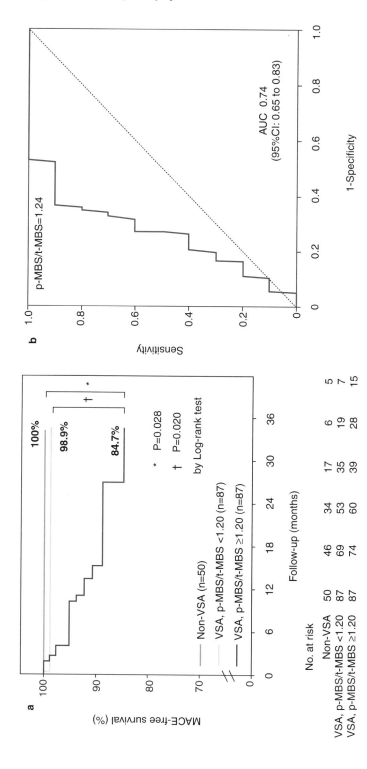

Fig. 3.6 Prognostic impact of Rho-kinase activity in circulating leukocytes in VSA patients. The Kaplan–Meier curve for cardiac events (cardiac death, non-fatal myocardial infarction, and hospitalization for unstable angina) of VSA patients with high Rho-kinase activity (≥1.20) *vs.* those with low Rho-kinase activity (<1.20) *vs.* non-VSA patients (**a**). ROC analysis for predicting future development of cardiac events of VSA patients confirmed that a p-MBS ratio of 1.24 was identified as the best cutoff level (**b**). (Reproduced from Nihei et al. [26])

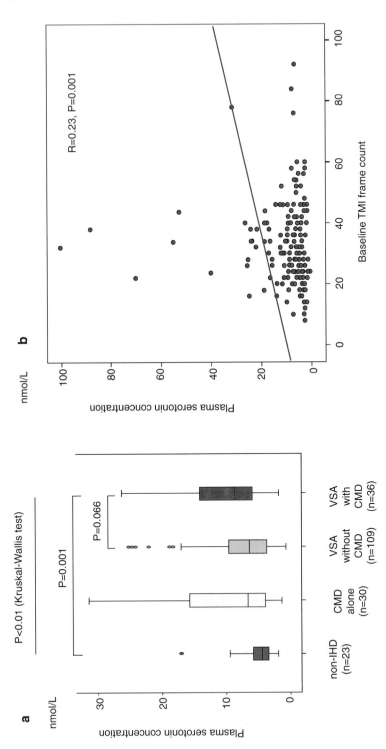

Fig. 3.7 Plasma serotonin concentration for discrimination of VSA patients with coronary microvascular dysfunction (CMD). Plasma concentrations of serotonin by patient group classified in accordance with the diagnosis of VSA with or without CMD (**a**). CMD was defined as myocardial lactate production despite the absence of angiographically demonstrable epicardial coronary spasm. Among the 4 patient groups, serotonin concentrations were highest in the VSA with CMD group. There was a positive correlation between TIMI (Thrombolysis In Myocardial Infarction) frame count, a marker of coronary vascular resistance, and plasma serotonin concentrations. (Reproduced from Odaka et al. [25])

measured plasma concentration of serotonin, and found that VSA patients with CMD had highest serotonin concentration, while no difference was noted between VSA and non-VSA groups, associated with increased coronary vascular resistance (Fig. 3.7) [31]. Fractional flow reserve (FFR), a marker for evaluating the degree of flow limiting coronary stenotic region, may also be able to extract the high-risk population among VSA patients [32].

3.5 Imaging for Coronary Artery Spasm

Cardiovascular imaging could offer additional information at cellular and molecular levels on the detailed features of VSA. Intravascular imaging studies reported that atherosclerotic changes are more common in the human coronary arterial segment of focal spasm as compared with that of diffuse spasm [33, 34]. We have previously demonstrated that chronic inflammatory changes in the coronary adventitia play important roles in the pathogenesis of coronary artery spasm through Rho-kinase activation and resultant vascular smooth muscle hypercontraction [35–37]. We thus sought to develop novel imaging approaches for evaluating the extent of coronary adventitial inflammatory changes in VSA patients in vivo. First, a mode of Fourier-domain (FD) optical coherence tomography (OCT) [38] is capable of visualizing a nutrient blood vessel for coronary arterial wall linking to the intima/media, termed adventitial vasa vasorum (VV) [39, 40] in pigs and humans ex vivo. In these studies, we used the definition of adventitial area as [area outside the external elastic lamina within a distance of the thickness of intima plus media—vessel area] and the definition of adventitial VV area density calculated by [adventitial VV area/adventitial area] [39]. We were able to demonstrate that OCT-delineated adventitial VV formation was significantly enhanced at the spastic segments of VSA patients as compared with those of control subjects (Fig. 3.8a–d) [41, 43]. Adventitial VV formation was significantly enhanced in the group with high JCSA score than in that with low or intermediate score. Second, coronary perivascular adipose tissue (PVAT) volume measured by CT coronary angiography was increased at the spastic segment of VSA patients [44]. Subsequently, ^{18}F-fluorodeoxyglucose (^{18}F-FDG) positron emission tomographic (PET) imaging allows us to evaluate inflammatory changes of coronary PVAT in pigs in vivo [42]. In this study, the extent of PVAT inflammation was expressed as target to background ratio (TBR), the standardized uptake value (SUV) corrected for blood activity by dividing the average blood SUV estimated from the ascending aorta. With the novel approach of ^{18}F-FDG PET, we demonstrated that coronary PVAT inflammatory changes were more extensive at the spastic coronary segments of VSA patients as compared with those of control subjects (Fig. 3.8e–i) [45]. Inflammatory changes measured by ^{18}F-FDG PET were significantly suppressed after medical treatment (Fig. 3.8j). These imaging approaches may serve as a promising avenue for the fully elucidation of the pathogenesis of coronary artery spasm in living patients with VSA in vivo.

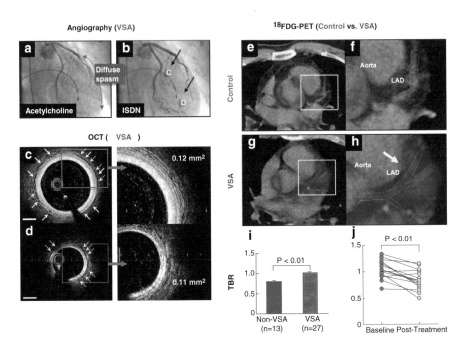

Fig. 3.8 Imaging of coronary artery spasm. Representative coronary angiography after administration of intracoronary acetylcholine (**a**), after resolving the spasm with intracoronary administration of isosorbide-dinitrate (ISDN) (**b**), and cross-sectional images of optical coherence tomography (OCT) of a VSA patient with provoked diffuse spams (**c**, **d**). After ISDN, the coronary artery was imaged by OCT (**b**), and adventitial vasa vasorum (VV) (yellow arrows) were manually segmented on each frame. Adventitial VV area was then calculated as shown in magnified OCT images. Scale bars: 1 mm (**c**, **d**). (Reprinted with permission from Nishimiya et al. [41]). Representative ¹⁸F-fluorodeoxyglucose (¹⁸F-FDG) positron emission tomographic (PET) images of a non-VSA control subject and a VSA patient (**e–h**), suggesting that coronary perivascular adipose tissue (PVAT) inflammation is markedly increased at the spastic segments of the left anterior descending coronary artery (LAD) of the VSA patient (**g**, **h**). Quantitative analysis showed that TBR in coronary PVAT measured at the spastic LAD was significantly greater in the VSA group than in the non-VSA control group (**i**). TBR was significantly decreased in the VSA group after medical treatment (**j**). (Reproduced from Ohyama et al. [42])

3.6 Future Perspectives

A recent large-scale trial has shown that the coronary intervention for myocardial ischemia related to organic stenosis ended up showing no significant improvement in exercise time when compared with a placebo procedure [46] and may not result in the risk reduction of future cardiovascular events [46–48]. These results emphasize in part the importance of the assessment of coronary vasomotion abnormalities, including coronary artery spasm (VSA), rather than stenosis-related myocardial ischemia (Fig. 3.9). In conclusions, we strongly encourage to perform spasm provocation tests even when no organic coronary stenosis is found angiographically, and expect to possess more sophisticated approaches that can be readily used in daily

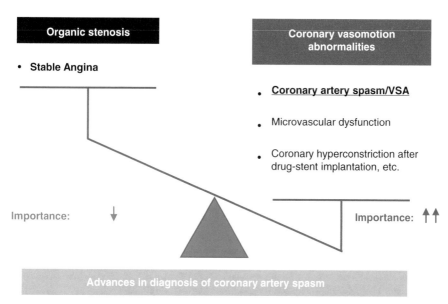

Fig. 3.9 Recent large scale cohorts have emphasized in part the importance of the assessment of coronary vasomotion abnormalities, including coronary artery spasm (VSA), rather than stenosis-related myocardial ischemia in patients with stable ischemic heart disease. This chapter highlighted recent advances in diagnostic methodology of coronary artery spasm

clinical practice, enabling us to predict the prevalence and the disease activity of VSA.

Acknowledgements We would like to thank Takashi Shiroto, MD, PhD, Ryuji Tsuburaya, MD, PhD, Kentaro Aizawa, MD, PhD, Yoku Kikuchi, MD, PhD, Yusuke Takagi, MD, PhD, Taro Nihei, MD, PhD, Yuji Odaka, MD, PhD, and Kazuma Ohyama, MD, PhD, for their contributions to the research works at the Department of Cardiovascular Medicine, Tohoku University Graduate School of Medicine.

Disclosure: None.

References

1. JCS joint working group. Guidelines for diagnosis and treatment of patients with vasospastic angina (coronary spastic angina). Circ J. 2014;78:2779–801. https://doi.org/10.1253/circj.CJ-66-0098.

2. Beltrame JF, Crea F, Kaski JC, Ogawa H, Ong P, Sechtem U, Shimokawa H, Bairey Merz CN, Coronary Vasomotion Disorders International Study Group (COVADIS). International standardization of diagnostic criteria for vasospastic angina. Eur Heart J. 2017;38:2565–8. https://doi.org/10.1093/eurheartj/ehv351.

3. Yasue H, Horio T, Nakamura N, Fujii H, Imoto N, Sonoda R, Kugiyama K, Obata K, Morikami Y, Kimura T. Induction of coronary artery spasm by acetylcholine in patients with variant angina: possible role of the parasympathetic nervous system in the pathogenesis of coronary artery spasm. Circulation. 1986;74:955–63. https://doi.org/10.1161/01.cir.74.5.955.

4. Okumura K, Yasue H, Matsuyama K, Goto K, Miyagi H, Ogawa H, Matsuyama K. Sensitivity and specificity of intracoronary injection of acetylcholine for the inductin of coronary artery spasm. J Am Coll Cardiol. 1988;12:883–8. https://doi.org/10.1016/0735-1097(88)90449-4.

5. Ong P, Athanasiadis A, Hill S, Vogelsberg H, Voehringer M, Sechtem U. Coronary artery spasm as a frequent cause of acute coronary syndrome. The CASPAR (coronary artery spasm in patients with acute coronary syndrome) study. J Am Coll Cardiol. 2008;52:523–7. https://doi.org/10.1016/j.jacc.2008.04.050.

6. Ong P, Athanasiadis A, Borgulya G, Vokshi I, Bastiaenen R, Kubik S, Hill S, Schäufele T, Mahrholdt H, Kaski JC, Sechtem U. Clinical usefulness, angiographic characteristics, and safety evaluation of intracoronary acetylcholine provocation testing among 921 consecutive white patients with unobstructed coronary arteries. Circulation. 2014;129:1723–30. https://doi.org/10.1161/CIRCULATIONAHA.113.004096.

7. Stein L. Observations on the action of ergonovine on the coronary circulation and its use in the diagnosis of coronary artery insufficiency. Am Heart J. 1949;39:36–45.

8. Heupler FA. Provocative testing for coronary arterial spasm: risk, method and rationale. Am J Cardiol. 1980;46:335–7. https://doi.org/10.1016/0002-9149(80)90081-8.

9. Curry RC, Pepine CJ, Sabom MB, Conti CR. Similarities of ergonovine-induced and spontaneous attacks of varian angina. Circulation. 1979;59:307–12. https://doi.org/10.1161/01.cir.59.2.307.

10. Shimokawa H. 2014 William Harvey lecture: importance of coronary vasomotion abnormalities - from bench to bedside. Eur Heart J. 2014;35:3180–93. https://doi.org/10.1093/eurheartj/ehu427.

11. Takagi Y, Yasuda S, Takahashi J, Tsunoda R, Ogata Y, Seki A, Sumiyoshi T, Matsui M, Goto T, Tanabe Y, Sueda S, Sato T, Ogawa S, Kubo N, Momomura S, Ogawa H, Shimokawa H, Japanese Coronary Spasm Association. Clinical implications of provocation tests for coronary artery spasm: safety, arrhythmic complications, and prognostic impact: multicenter registry study of the Japanese Coronary Spasm Association. Eur Heart J. 2013;34:258–67. https://doi.org/10.1093/eurheartj/ehs199.

12. Takagi Y, Takahashi J, Yasuda S, Miyata S, Tsunoda R, Ogata Y, Seki A, Sumiyoshi T, Matsui M, Goto T, Tanabe Y, Sueda S, Sato T, Ogawa S, Kubo N, Momomura S, Ogawa H, Shimokawa H, Japanese Coronary Spasm Association. Prognostic stratification of patients with vasospastic angina: a comprehensive clinical risk score developed by the Japanese Coronary Spasm Association. J Am Coll Cardiol. 2013;62:1144–53. https://doi.org/10.1016/j.jacc.2013.07.018.

13. Pristipino C, Beltrame JF, Finocchiaro ML, Hattori R, Fujita M, Mongiardo R, Cianflone D, Sanna T, Sasayama S, Maseri A. Major racial differences in coronary constrictor response between Japanese and Caucasians with recent myocardial infarction. Circulation. 2000;101:1102–8. https://doi.org/10.1161/01.cir.101.10.1102.

14. Sato K, Takahashi J, Odaka Y, Suda A, Sueda S, Teragawa H, Ishii K, Kiyooka T, Hirayama A, Sumiyoshi T, Tanabe Y, Kimura K, Kaikita K, Ong P, Sechtem U, Camici PG, Kaski JC, Crea F, Beltrame JF, Shimokawa H, Japanese Coronary Spasm Association. Clinical characteristics and long-term prognosis of contemporary patients with vasospastic angina. Ethnic differences detected in an international comparative study. Int J Cardiol. 2019;291:13–8. https://doi.org/10.1016/j.ijcard.2019.02.038.

15. Shiroto T, Yasuda S, Tsuburaya R, Ito Y, Takahashi J, Ito K, Ishibashi-Ueda H, Shimokawa H. Role of Rho-kinase in the pathogenesis of coronary hyperconstricting responses induced

by drug-eluting stents in pigs in vivo. J Am Coll Cardiol. 2009;54:2321–9. https://doi.org/10.1016/j.jacc.2009.07.045.

16. Aizawa K, Yasuda S, Takahashi J, Takii T, Kikuchi Y, Tsuburaya R, Ito Y, Ito K, Nakayama M, Takeda M, Shimokawa H. Involvement of Rho-kinase activation in the pathogenesis of coronary hyperconstricting responses induced by drug-eluting stents in patients with coronary artery disease. Circ J. 2012;76:2552–60. https://doi.org/10.1253/circj.CJ-12-0662.

17. Tsuburaya R, Takahashi J, Nakamura A, Nozaki E, Sugi M, Yamamoto Y, Hiramoto T, Horiguchi S, Inoue K, Goto T, Kato A, Shinozaki T, Ishida E, Miyata S, Yasuda S, Shimokawa H, Investigators NOVEL. Beneficial effects of long-acting nifedipine on coronary vasomotion abnormalities after drug-eluting stent implantation: the NOVEL study. Eur Heart J. 2016;37:2713–21. https://doi.org/10.1093/eurheartj/ehw256.

18. Nishimiya K, Matsumoto Y, Uzuka H, Ogata T, Hirano M, Shindo T, Hasebe Y, Tsuburaya R, Shiroto T, Takahashi J, Ito K, Shimokawa H. Beneficial effects of a novel bioabsorbable polymer coating on enhanced coronary vasoconstricting responses after drug-eluting stent implantation in pigs in vivo. J Am Coll Cardiol Intv. 2016;9:281–91. https://doi.org/10.1016/j.jcin.2015.09.041.

19. Crea F, Bairey Merz CN, Beltrame JF, Berry C, Camici PG, Kaski JC, Ong P, Pepine CJ, Sechtem U, Shimokawa H. Mechanisms and diagnostic evaluation of persistent or recurrent angina following percutaneous coronary revascularization. Eur Heart J. 2019;40:2455–62. https://doi.org/10.1093/eurheartj/ehy857.

20. Mohri M, Koyanagi M, Egashira K, Tagawa H, Ichiki T, Shimokawa H, Takeshita A. Angina pectoris caused by coronary microvascular spasm. Lancet. 1998;351:1165–9. https://doi.org/10.1016/S0140-6736(97)07329-7.

21. Shimokawa H, Toyoda K, Matsumoto T, Sato H, Kikuchi Y, Nakamura M. Human leucocyte antigen and coronary artery spasm. Int J Cardiol. 1986;12:362–5.

22. Hizume T, Morikawa K, Takaki A, Abe K, Sunagawa K, Amano M, Kaibuchi K, Kubo C, Shimokawa H. Sustained elevation of serum cortisol level causes sensitization of coronary vasoconstricting responses in pigs in vivo. A possible link between stress and coronary vasospasm. Circ Res. 2006;99:767–75. https://doi.org/10.1161/01.RES.0000244093.69985.2f.

23. Kikuchi Y, Yasuda S, Aizawa K, Tsuburaya R, Ito Y, Takeda M, Nakayama M, Ito K, Takahashi J, Shimokawa H. Enhanced Rho-kinase activity in circulating neutrophils of patients with vasospastic angina. A possible biomarker for diagnosis and disease activity assessment. J Am Coll Cardiol. 2011;58:1231–7. https://doi.org/10.1016/j.jacc.2011.05.046.

24. Nihei T, Takahashi J, Kikuchi Y, Takagi Y, Hao K, Tsuburaya R, Shiroto T, Ito Y, Matsumoto Y, Nakayama M, Ito K, Yasuda S, Shimokawa H. Enhanced Rho-kinase activity in patients with vasospastic angina after the Great East Japan earthquake. Circ J. 2012;76:2892–4. https://doi.org/10.1016/j.jacc.2011.05.046.

25. Nihei T, Kikuchi Y, Tsuburaya R, Ito Y, Shiroto T, Hao K, Takagi Y, Matsumoto Y, Nakayama M, Miyata S, Sakata Y, Ito K, Shimokawa H. Circadian variation of Rho-kinase activity in circulating leukocytes of patients with vasospastic angina. Circ J. 2014;78:1183–90. https://doi.org/10.1253/circj.CJ-13-1458.

26. Nihei T, Takahashi J, Hao K, Kikuchi Y, Odaka Y, Tsuburaya R, Nishimiya K, Matsumoto Y, Ito K, Miyata S, Sakata Y, Shimokawa H. Prognostic impacts of Rho-kinase activity in circulating leukocytes in patients with vasospastic angina. Eur Heart J. 2018;39:952–9. https://doi.org/10.1093/eurheartj/ehx657.

27. Ong P, Camici PG, Beltrame JF, Crea F, Shimokawa H, Sechtem U, Kaski JC, Bairey Merz CN, Coronary Vasomotion Disorders International Study Group (COVADIS). International standardization of diagnostic criteria for microvascular angina. Int J Cardiol. 2018;250:16–20. https://doi.org/10.1016/j.ijcard.2017.08.068.

28. Bairey Merz CN, Pepine CJ, Walsh MN, Fleg JL. Ischemia and no obstructive coronary artery disease (INOCA). Developing evidence-based therapies and research agenda for the next decade. Circulation. 2017;135:1075–92. https://doi.org/10.1161/CIRCULATIONAHA.116.024534.

29. Kobayashi Y, Fearon WF, Honda Y, Tanaka S, Pargaonkar V, Fitzgerald PJ, Lee DP, Stefanick M, Yeung AC, Tremmel JA. Effect of sex differences on invasive measures of coronary macrovascular dysfunction in patients with angina in the absence of obstructive coronary artery disease. J Am Coll Cardiol Intv. 2015;8:1433–41. https://doi.org/10.1016/j.jcin.2015.03.045.

30. Suda A, Takahashi J, Hao K, Kikuchi Y, Shindo T, Ikeda S, Sato K, Sugisawa J, Matsumoto Y, Miyata S, Sakata Y, Shimokawa H. Coronary functional abnormalities in patients with angina and nonobstructive coronary artery disease. J Am Coll Cardiol. 2019;74:2350–60. https://doi.org/10.1016/j.jacc.2019.08.1056.

31. Odaka Y, Takahashi J, Tsuburaya R, Nishimiya K, Hao K, Matsumoto Y, Ito K, Sakata Y, Miyata S, Manita D, Hirowatari Y, Shimokawa H. Plasma concentration of serotonin is a novel biomarker for coronary microvascular dysfunction in patients with suspected angina and unbstructive coronary arteries. Eur Heart J. 2017;38:489–96. https://doi.org/10.1093/eurheartj/ehw448.

32. Hao K, Takahashi J, Suda A, Sato K, Sugisawa J, Tsuchiya S, Shindo T, Ikeda S, Kikuchi Y, Shiroto T, Matsumoto Y, Sakata Y, Shimokawa H. Clinical importance of fractional flow reserve in patients with organic coronary stenosis and vasospastic angina. Eur Heart J. 2019;40(Supplement_1). https://doi.org/10.1093/eurheartj/ehz745.0436.

33. Koyama J, Yamaghisi M, Tamai J, Tamai J, Kawano S, Daikoku S, Miyatake K. Comparison of vessel wall morphologic appearance at sits of focal and diffuse coronary vasospasm by intravascular ultrasound. Am Heart J. 1995;130:440–5. https://doi.org/10.1016/0002-8703(95)90349-6.

34. Kitano D, Takayama T, Sudo M, Kogo T, Kojima K, Akutsu N, Nishida T, Haruta H, Fukamachi D, Kawano T, Kanai T, Hiro T, Saito S, Hirayma A. Angioscopic differences of coronary intima between diffuse and focal coronary vasospasm: comparison of optical coherence tomography findings. J Cardiol. 2018;72:200–7. https://doi.org/10.1016/j.jjcc.2018.04.013.

35. Shimokawa H, Ito A, Fulumoto Y, Kadokami T, Nakaike R, Sakata M, Takayanagi T, Egashira K, Takeshita A. Chronic treatment with interluekin-1β induces coronary intimal lesions and vasospastic responses in pigs in vivo. The role of platelet-derived growth factor. J Clin Invest. 1996;97:769–76. https://doi.org/10.1172/JCI118476.

36. Kandabashi T, Shimokawa H, Miyata K, Kunihiro I, Kawano Y, Fukata Y, Higo T, Egashira K, Takahashi S, Kaibuchi K, Takeshita A. Inhibition of myosin phosphatase by upregulated Rho-kinase plays a key role for coronary artery spasm in a porcine model with interleukin-1β. Eur Heart J. 2017;38:489–96. https://doi.org/10.1161/01.cir.101.11.1319.

37. Masumoto A, Mohri M, Shimokawa H, Urakami L, Usui M, Takeshita A. Suppression of coronary artery spasm by the Rho-kinase inhibitor fasudil in patients with vasospastic angina. Circulation. 2002;105:1545–7. https://doi.org/10.1161/hc1002.105938.

38. Yun SH, Tearney GJ, Vakoc BJ, Shishkov M, Oh WY, Desjardins AE, Suter MJ, Chan RC, Evans JA, Jang IK, Nishioka NS, de Boer JF, Bouma BE. Comprehensive volumetric optical microscopy in vivo. Nat Med. 2006;12:1429–33. https://doi.org/10.1038/nm1450.

39. Nishimiya K, Matsumoto Y, Takahashi J, Uzuka H, Odaka Y, Nihei T, Hao K, Tsuburaya R, Ito K, Shimokawa H. In vivo visualization of adventitial vasa vasorum of the human coronary artery on optical frequency domain imaging. Validation study. Circ J. 2014;78:2516–8. https://doi.org/10.1253/circj.CJ-14-0485.

40. Nishimiya K, Matsumoto Y, Uzuka H, Oyama K, Tanaka A, Taruya A, Ogata T, Hirano M, Shindo T, Hanawa K, Hasebe Y, Hao K, Tsuburaya R, Takahashi J, Miyata S, Ito K, Akasaka T, Shimokawa H. Accuracy of optical frequency domain imaging for evaluation of coronary adventitial vasa vasorum formation after stent implantation in pigs and humans. A validation study. Circ J. 2015;79:1323–31. https://doi.org/10.1253/circj.CJ-15-0078.

41. Nishimiya K, Matsumoto Y, Uzuka H, Ohyama K, Hao K, Tsuburaya R, Shiroto T, Takahashi J, Ito K, Shimokawa H. Focal vasa vasorum formation in patients with focal coronary vasospasm. -An optical frequency domain imaging study. Circ J. 2016;80:2252–4. https://doi.org/10.1253/circj.CJ-16-0580.

42. Ohyama K, Matsumoto Y, Amamizu H, Uzuka H, Nishimiya K, Morosawa S, Hirano M, Watabe H, Funaki Y, Miyata S, Takahashi J, Ito K, Shimokawa H. Association of coronary perivascular adipose tissue inflammation and DES-induced coronary hyperconstriction responses in pigs. -^{18}F-FDG PET imaging study. Arterior Thromb Vasc Biol. 2017;37:1757–64. https://doi.org/10.1161/atvbaha.117.309843.

43. Nishimiya K, Matsumoto Y, Takahashi J, Uzuka H, Wang H, Tsuburaya R, Hao K, Ohyama K, Odaka Y, Miyata S, Ito K, Shimokawa H. Enhanced adventitial vasa vasorum formation in patients with vasospastic angina. J Am Coll Cardiol. 2016;67:598–600. https://doi.org/10.1016/j.jacc.2015.11.031.

44. Ohyama K, Matsumoto Y, Nishimiya K, Hao K, Tsuburaya R, Ota H, Amamizu H, Uzuka H, Takahashi J, Ito K, Shimokawa H. Increased coronary perivascular adipose tissue volume in patients with vasospastic angina. Circ J. 2016;80:1653–6. https://doi.org/10.1253/circj.CJ-16-0213.

45. Ohyama K, Matsumoto Y, Takanami K, Ota H, Nishimiya K, Sugisawa J, Tsuchiya S, Amamizu H, Uzuka H, Suda A, Shindo T, Kikuchi Y, Hao K, Tsuburaya R, Takahashi J, Miyata S, Sakata Y, Takase K, Shimokawa H. Coronary adventitial and perivascular adipose tissue inflammation in patients with vasospastic angina. J Am Coll Cardiol. 2018;71:414–25. https://doi.org/10.1016/j.jacc.2017.11.046.

46. Al-Lamee R, Thompson D, Dehbi HM, Sen S, Tang K, Davies J, Keeble T, Mielewczik M, Kaprielian R, Malik IS, Nijjer SS, Petraco R, Cook C, Ahmad Y, Howard J, Baker C, Sharp A, Gerber R, Talwar S, Assomull R, Mayet J, Wensel R, Collier D, Shun-Shin M, Thom SA, Davies JE, Francis DP, ORBITA investigators. Percutaneous coronary intervention in stable angina (ORBITA): a double-blind, randomised controlled trial. Lancet. 2018;391:31–40. https://doi.org/10.1016/S0140-6736(17)32714-9.

47. Boden WE, O'Rourke RA, Teo KK, Hartigan PM, Maron DJ, Kostuk WJ, Knudtson M, Dada M, Casperson P, Harris CL, Chaitman BR, Shaw L, Gosselin G, Nawaz S, Title LM, Gau G, Blaustein AS, Booth DC, Bates ER, Spertus JA, Berman DS, Mancini GB, Weintraub WS, COURAGE Trial Research Group. Optimal medical therapy with or without PCI for stable coronary disease. N Engl J Med. 2007;356:1503–16. https://doi.org/10.1056/NEJMoa070829.

48. Maron DJ, Hochman JS, Reynolds HR, Bangalore S, O'Brien SM, Boden WE, Chaitman BR, Senior R, López-Sendón J, Alexander KP, Lopes RD, Shaw LJ, Berger JS, Newman JD, Sidhu MS, Goodman SG, Ruzyllo W, Gosselin G, Maggioni AP, White HD, Bhargava B, Min JK, GBJ M, Berman DS, Picard MH, Kwong RY, Ali ZA, Mark DB, Spertus JA, Krishnan MN, Elghamaz A, Moorthy N, Hueb WA, Demkow M, Mavromatis K, Bockeria O, Peteiro J, Miller TD, Szwed H, Doerr R, Keltai M, Selvanayagam JB, Steg PG, Held C, Kohsaka S, Mavromichalis S, Kirby R, Jeffries NO, Harrell FE Jr, Rockhold FW, Broderick S, Ferguson TB Jr, Williams DO, Harrington RA, Stone GW, Rosenberg Y, ISCHEMIA Research Group. Initial invasive or conservative strategy for stable coronary disease. N Engl J Med. 2020;382:1395–407. https://doi.org/10.1056/NEJMoa1915922.

Chapter 4
Treatment of Coronary Artery Spasm

Yasuharu Matsumoto, Kensuke Nishimiya, Kazuma Ohyama, Hironori Uzuka, Hirokazu Amamizu, Jun Takahashi, and Hiroaki Shimokawa

Abstract Coronary artery spasm plays a key role in a wide range of ischemic heart diseases not only in vasospastic angina (VSA) but also in acute coronary syndrome and sudden cardiac death in Asia and Western countries. In the era of widespread utilization of drug-eluting stents (DES) in the field of coronary intervention, it is important to realize the fact that patients still have unremitting angina symptoms even after resolving organic coronary stenosis with DES implantation. Although conventional management of VSA involves lifestyle modifications, use of established pharmacological therapies, further novel therapies need to be developed. Basic and clinical evidence also has been accumulated for elucidating the risk to predict future cardiovascular events, detailed mechanism of coronary artery spasm, which in turn, provides new therapeutic approach for coronary spasm. In this chapter, we will summarize the recent advances in the treatment of coronary artery spasm mainly based on our findings.

Keywords Coronary artery spasm · Vasospastic angina · Life style · Calcium channel blockers · Nitrates · Rho-Kinase inhibitors · Fasudil · Inflammation

Y. Matsumoto · K. Nishimiya · K. Ohyama · H. Uzuka · H. Amamizu · J. Takahashi · H. Shimokawa (✉)
Department of Cardiovascular Medicine, Tohoku University Graduate School of Medicine, Sendai, Miyagi, Japan
e-mail: shimo@cardio.med.tohoku.ac.jp

4.1   Importance of Treatment of Coronary Artery Spasm Worldwide

Coronary artery spasm plays an important role in a wide variety of ischemic heart disease, not only in VSA but also in other forms of angina pectoris, myocardial infarction, and sudden death [1]. Although it has been believed for a long time that VSA is more common in Asian than in Western populations [2, 3], recent studies from Germany revealed that the prevalence of VSA in Caucasians may be higher than what we expected [4, 5]. We also have recently addressed the ethnic differences in the long-term prognosis by comparing 1339 Japanese and 118 Caucasians VSA patients [6]. Multivessel spasm was more prevalent in Japanese, whereas provocation-related arrhythmias were more common in Caucasians. In the multi-variable analysis, the Japanese Coronary Spasm Association (JCSA) risk score, including the number of coronary arteries positive for spasm provocation tests, was found to show good correlations with major adverse cardiac event (MACE) rates in both Japanese and Caucasian patients. Thus, these findings indicate the clinical importance of the treatment of VSA worldwide.

4.2   Management of Coronary Artery spasm

Management of VSA includes lifestyle modifications, use of pharmacological therapies, and non-pharmacological approaches [1, 7]. It is important to document suppression of both symptomatic and asymptomatic episodes with ambulatory ECG monitoring [7]. Risk stratification of future cardiovascular events in VSA patients is also important [8]. Treatment of VSA reduces the frequency of symptomatic episodes and appears to decrease the frequency of serious complications [7]. Associated with decreased disease activity and symptoms, biomarkers and cardiac images are also useful [9, 10].

4.2.1   Lifestyle Modifications for Risk Factors

We previously demonstrated that inflammatory stimuli causes upregulation of Rho-kinase leading to coronary artery spasm [11]. Notably, cigarette smoking has been shown to cause low-grade inflammation [12], which may also cause coronary spasm. Since smoking cessation removes one of the triggers for VSA and leads to a significant decrease in the frequency of episodes, at least in a short term, it should be encouraged [13]. Avoiding other risk factors for VSA, such as mental stress [14], alcohol consumption [15], and the use of pharmacological agents, such as cocaine [16], is also important in VSA patients. Indeed, we previously demonstrated that sustained elevation of serum cortisol level sensitizes coronary arteries to cause hyperconstricting responses through Rho-kinase activation in pigs in vivo, suggesting the link between stress and coronary artery spasm [17].

4.2.2 Pharmacotherapy

Calcium Channel Blockers

Calcium channel blockers (CCBs) are the first-line therapy for VSA [7]. Indeed, CCBs effectively inhibit vasoconstriction and promote vasodilation of the coronary vasculature, thereby alleviating symptoms. Previous study demonstrated that the use of CCBs was an independent predictor of myocardial infarct-free survival in VSA patients [18].

In the era of coronary intervention with DES, it is important to realize the fact that patients have unremitting angina symptoms even after resolving organic coronary stenosis with DES implantation [19]. We have demonstrated that a first-generation DES cause coronary hyperconstricting responses in pigs in vivo in response to intracoronary serotonin at the segments proximal or distal to the DES edge, compared with its platform bare-metal stents (BMS) and that activation of Rho-kinase pathway, a molecular switch for vascular smooth muscle contraction, is involved in its pathogenesis [20]. More recently, we conducted a multicenter randomized control study that showed that even the everolimus-eluting stents, most widely disseminated DES, were able to induce coronary hyperconstricting responses at 8–10 months after DES implantation [21]. Intriguingly, nifedipine, a long-acting CCB, was able to suppress DES-induced coronary hyperconstricting responses in humans [21]. We and others also demonstrated that among the 4 major CCBs (benidipine, amlodipine, nifedipine, and diltiazem) that effectively suppress VSA attacks in general, benidipine showed the most beneficial prognostic effects than others [22, 23]. Taken together, CCBs are useful for the treatment of VSA patients with or without DES implantation.

Nitrates and Nicorandil

Long-acting nitrates are also effective in alleviating symptoms [7], although the potential nitrate tolerance makes them a less desirable first-line approach. Indeed, we addressed this important issue on the long-term efficacy of nitrate therapy in VSA patients [24]. In this study with 1429 patients with VSA, of whom more than 90 percent were receiving treatment with a CCB, a propensity score-matched analysis found that the cumulative incidence of MACE (cardiac death, nonfatal myocardial infarction, hospitalization due to unstable angina or heart failure, and appropriate implantable cardioverter-defibrillator shocks) was similar between patients with nitrate treatment and those without it (11 vs. 8% at 5 years; hazard ratio [HR] 1.28,

95% CI 0.72–2.28) [24]. Although nicorandil, one of the nitrate-like agents used in the study, had a neutral effect on clinical events (HR: 0.80; 95% CI 0.28–2.27), multivariable analysis showed a deleterious effect of the concomitant use of nitrates and nicorandil (HR 2.14; 95% CI 1.02–4.47). Thus, the long-term administration of nitrates may not improve prognosis in VSA patients who receive CCB treatment. In addition, the concomitant use of more than one nitrate formulation may increase the risk for MACE in those patients.

Rho-Kinase Inhibitors

Accumulating evidence indicates that Rho-kinase is substantially involved in the pathogenesis of coronary spasm in animals and in humans [1]. Indeed, intracoronary administration of fasudil and of hydroxyfasudil, selective Rho-kinase inhibitors, markedly inhibits coronary spasm in a porcine model with long-term treatment with IL-1β [25–27]. Importantly, the inhibition of Rho-kinase with fasudil/hydroxyfasudil was associated with the suppression of enhanced MLC phosphorylations (both MLC mono- and diphosphorylations) at the spastic coronary segments in this model [25, 26]. Subsequently, it was demonstrated that the expression and activity of Rho-kinase are enhanced at the IL-1β-induced inflammatory coronary lesions, thereby suppressing MLCPh through phosphorylation of its MBS with resultant increase in MLC phosphorylations and coronary spasm [28]. This is also the case for the hypercontractions of isolated arteriosclerotic human arteries [29].

We then demonstrated that in VSA patients, intracoronary fasudil also markedly inhibits acetylcholine-induced coronary spasm and related myocardial ischemia, demonstrating that Rho-kinase is substantially involved in the pathogenesis of coronary spasm in humans (Fig. 4.1) [30]. Severe coronary artery spasm after coronary artery bypass grafting (CABG) remains a serious complication of the surgery as it eventually results in circulatory collapse and/or death [31]. We also showed that the treatment with fasudil is useful to treat intractable and otherwise fatal coronary spasm resistant to intensive conventional vasodilator therapy after CABG (Fig. 4.2) [32]. We further conducted a clinical trial for anti-anginal effects of fasudil in patients with stable effort angina, which demonstrated that the long-term oral treatment with the Rho-kinase inhibitor is effective in ameliorating exercise tolerance in patients with adequate safety profiles [33]. Approximately half of VSA patients show abnormal responses to exercise stress tests [34]. These findings suggest that inappropriate coronary vasoconstriction may be involved even in the pathogenesis of effort angina that is effectively suppressed by Rho-kinase inhibitors.

DES-induced coronary vasomotion abnormalities even after successful PCI remains to be overcome [19]. We experienced a patient who suffered from an out-of-hospital cardiac arrest at 65 months after a sirolimus-eluting stent (first-generation DES) implantation [35]. Spasm provocation test using acetylcholine showed coronary spasm at the DES edges, whereas intracoronary pretreatment of Rho-kinase inhibitor, fasudil, markedly attenuated acetylcholine-induced vasoconstriction [35]. We also demonstrated that pretreatment with fasudil suppresses

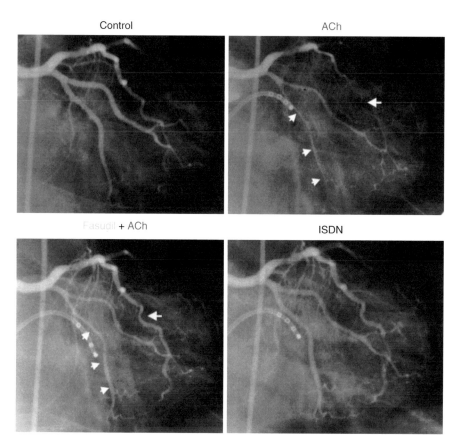

Fig. 4.1 Inhibitory effect of fasudil on coronary artery spasm. Top left, Baseline angiogram. Top right, The first ACh challenge provoked severe coronary spasm at the mid-portion of the left anterior descending coronary artery (large arrow) and diffuse spasm along the left circumflex coronary artery (small arrows). Bottom left, No epicardial spasm was provoked during the second challenge after pretreatment with fasudil. Bottom right, Angiogram after treatment with intracoronary isosorbide dinitrate (ISDN). (Reproduced from Masumoto et al. [30])

acetylcholine-induced coronary hyperconstricting responses in patients with DES implantation (Fig. 4.3) [36]. Taken together, Rho-kinase inhibitors are effective and promising drugs for the treatment of coronary artery spasm [1, 7].

Statins and Magnesium

In 64 patients who received CCB therapy, the percentage of ACh-induced coronary spasm was significantly lower in the group who received fluvastatin (30 mg/day) compared with those without it (48 vs. 79%) [37]. Magnesium deficiency may also play a role in coronary artery spasm [38]. In the previous study with 22 VSA patients, those who received intravenous magnesium ($n = 14$) showed coronary

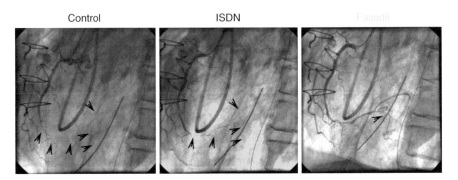

Fig. 4.2 Inhibitory effect of fasudil on intractable coronary spasm after CABG. Right coronary angiography of a patient with intractable coronary spasm after CABG. Black arrows indicate the spastic segments. Control, ISDN, and Fasudil indicate angiograms under control conditions, after intracoronary administration of isosorbide dinitrate (ISDN), and after fasudil, respectively. (Reproduced from Inokuchi et al. [32])

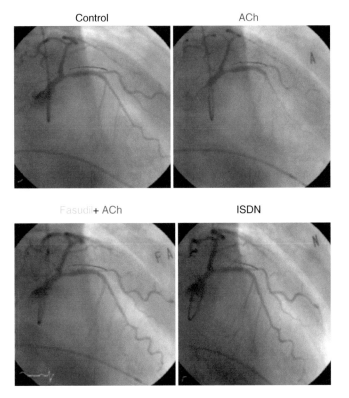

Fig. 4.3 Inhibitory effect of fasudil on drug-eluting stent-induced coronary hyperconstricting responses. *Top left*, Baseline angiogram. *Top right*, The first ACh challenge provoked severe coronary spasm at the mid-portion of the left anterior descending coronary artery (large arrow) and diffuse spasm along the left circumflex coronary artery (small arrows). *Bottom left*, No epicardial spasm was provoked during the second challenge after pretreatment with fasudil. *Bottom right*, Angiogram after treatment with intracoronary isosorbide dinitrate (ISDN). Red lines indicate the site of first-generation drug-eluting stent (Cypher™) implantation. (Reproduced from Aizawa et al. [36])

vasodilation compared with those with placebo ($n = 8$) [39]. Rechallenged intracoronary acetylcholine provocation tests also showed that they had less severe chest pain and ST-segment elevation. Further large studies are required to assess clinical outcomes before we recommend routine use of statins or magnesium for VSA patients.

4.2.3 Non-pharmacological Treatment

Novel non-pharmacological management of coronary vasomotion abnormalities includes, as we have recently demonstrated, catheter-based renal denervation (RDN) [40], improvement of DES polymers [41], exercise training [42], and a noninvasive low-intensity pulsed ultrasound (LIPUS) therapy [43].

The adventitia harbors a variety of components that potently modulate vascular tone, including sympathetic nerve fibers (SNF) and vasa vasorum [40]. Catheter-based RDN inhibits sympathetic nerve activity. Thus, we examined whether RDN suppresses drug-eluting stent-induced coronary hyperconstricting responses, and if so, what mechanisms are involved [40]. Pigs implanted with everolimus-eluting stents were randomly assigned to the RDN or sham group. The RDN group underwent renal ablation. At 1 month, RDN significantly caused marked damage of the SNF at the renal arteries without any stenosis, thrombus, or dissections. Notably, RDN significantly upregulated the expression of α_2-adrenergic receptor-binding sites in the nucleus tractus solitaries of the brain stem, attenuated muscle sympathetic nerve activity, and decreased systolic blood pressure and plasma renin activity. In addition, RDN attenuated coronary hyperconstricting responses to intracoronary serotonin at the proximal and distal stent edges associated with decreases in SNF and vasa vasorum formation, inflammatory cell infiltration, and Rho-kinase expression/activation. Furthermore, there were significant positive correlations between SNF and vasa vasorum and between SNF and coronary vasoconstricting responses. These results provide the first direct evidence that RDN ameliorates drug-eluting stent-induced coronary hyperconstricting responses in pigs in vivo through the kidney–brain–heart axis (Fig. 4.4) [40].

Recent studies have reported unremitting angina due to coronary vasomotion abnormalities even after successful DES implantation [19]. However, it remains to be elucidated which component of DES (metal stent, polymer coating, or antiproliferative drug) is responsible for DES-induced coronary hyperconstricting responses. We developed poly-dl-lactic acid and polycaprolactone (PDLLA-PCL) copolymer technology with higher biocompatibility that is resorbed within 3 months [41]. Four types of coronary stents were made; (1) a stent with polylactic acid (PLA) polymer coating containing antiproliferative drug (P1+ D+), (2) a stent with PLA polymer coating alone without any drug (P1+ D−), (3) a stent with novel PDLLA-PCL polymer coating alone (P2+ D−), and (4) a bare-metal stent (P−D−). These 4 stents were randomly deployed in the left anterior descending and left circumflex coronary arteries in 12 pigs. After 1 month, coronary vasoconstriction in response to

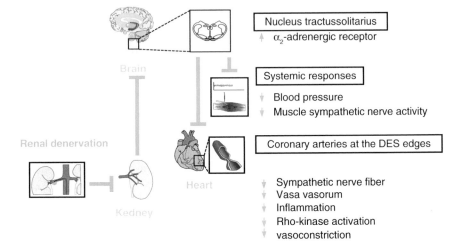

Fig. 4.4 Renal denervation as a potential novel therapeutic option for refractory coronary artery spasm. Bilateral renal denervation (RDN) ameliorates coronary hyperconstricting responses after DES implantation in pigs in vivo through suppression of the kidney–brain–heart axis, including suppressions of coronary adventitial sympathetic nerve fiber, vasa vasorum formation, inflammation, and Rho-kinase activation, suggesting that RDN is a novel therapeutic option for refractory angina. (Reproduced from Uzuka et al. [40])

intracoronary serotonin was enhanced at P1+ D+ and P1+ D− stent edges compared with P2+ D− and P−D− stent edges and was prevented by a specific Rho-kinase (a central molecule of coronary spasm) inhibitor, hydroxyfasudil. Immunostainings showed that inflammatory changes and Rho-kinase activation were significantly enhanced at P1+ D+ and P1+ D− sites compared with P2+ D− and P−D− sites. There were significant positive correlations between the extent of inflammation or Rho-kinase expression/activation and that of coronary vasoconstriction. These results indicate the causative roles of PLA polymer coating in DES-induced coronary vasoconstricting responses through inflammatory changes and Rho-kinase activation in pigs in vivo, which could be ameliorated by PDLLA-PCL copolymers (Fig. 4.5) [41].

Coronary vasomotion abnormalities could develop in both epicardial coronary arteries and intramuscular coronary microvessels. We thus examined whether vasodilator capacity of coronary microvessels is impaired in VSA patients and if so, whether exercise training could ameliorate vasodilator capacity of coronary microvessels, exercise tolerance, and angina symptoms on the top of CCB. Exercise training is effective for VSA patients in terms of improved vasodilator capacity of coronary microvessels, exercise tolerance, and angina symptoms even on the top of CCB [42].

However, a direct therapeutic approach to the coronary adventitia remains to be developed. We have developed a noninvasive, low-intensity pulsed ultrasound (LIPUS) therapy for angina, which exerts angiogenic and anti-inflammatory effects

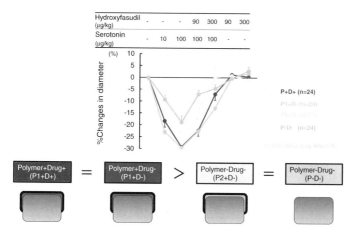

Fig. 4.5 Inhibitory effect of a novel polymer coating on coronary vasoconstricting responses at 1 month after stent implantation in pigs in vivo. Results of quantitative coronary angiography for coronary vasoconstricting response to serotonin (10 and 100 μg/kg IC) before and after hydroxyfasudil (90 and 300 μg/kg IC) at 1 month after stent implantation. Coronary vasoconstricting responses to serotonin were equally enhanced at the P1 + D+ and P1 + D− stent edges compared with the P2 + D− and P − D− stent edges. These responses were all prevented by pretreatment with hydroxyfasudil. The 4 different stents, P1 + D+, P1 + D−, P2 + D−, and P − D− (6 each), were randomly implanted in the LAD and LCX in 12 miniature pigs. At 1 month after stent implantation, animals underwent follow-up coronary angiography to assess coronary vasomotion in vivo and were then euthanized for histological and immunohistological analyses of the inflammation and expression/activity of Rho-kinase. IC = intracoronary; LAD = left anterior descending coronary artery; LCX = left circumflex coronary artery; P − D− = stent without a polymer or a drug; P1 + D+ = stent with a polylactic acid polymer and a drug; P1 + D− = stent with a polylactic acid polymer but without a drug; P2 + D− stent with a poly-dl-lactic acid and polycaprolactone copolymer but without a drug; PDLLA-PCL = poly-dl-lactic acid and polycaprolactone; PLA = polylactic acid. Results are expressed as mean ± SEM. (Reproduced from Nishimiya et al. [41])

through improved coronary microcirculation. We were able to develop a noninvasive LIPUS therapy for coronary functional abnormalities caused by chronic adventitial inflammation in pigs in vivo [43].

Percutaneous coronary intervention (PCI) is not routinely indicated for patients with focal spasm and minimal obstructive disease [7]. Coronary artery spasm and lethal ventricular arrhythmias are important causes of out-of-hospital cardiac arrest (OHCA) [44]. Optimal therapy for patients resuscitated from OHCA who are not found to have structural heart disease remains to be established. In 47 consecutive OHCA survivors without structural heart disease who had fully recovered (M/F 44/3, 43 ± 13 years), we performed dual induction tests, including acetylcholine provocation test first followed by programmed ventricular stimulation after 1–2 weeks. Patients with positive coronary spasm were treated with CCB-based anti-anginal medications, and implantable cardioverter-defibrillators (ICDs) were implanted in all patients [44]. Among OHCA survivors without structural heart disease, provokable coronary spasm and ventricular arrhythmias are common and can be seen in Brugada syndrome. No ventricular fibrillation episodes were noted in the spasm-alone patients who did not also have Brugada syndrome. Thus, patients with coronary spasm alone without Brugada syndrome may be a lower-risk group [44]. Importantly, placement of an ICD was not associated with improved survival in patients with variant angina and OHCA [45]. Thus, although there are no current guidelines for patients with VSA among OHCA survivors, an ICD should be considered based on the presence or absence of Brugada syndrome [44].

4.3   Usefulness of JCSA Risk Score for Risk Stratification of Future Cardiovascular Events

A landmark study from the JCSA registry developed the JCSA risk score that can provide comprehensive risk assessment and prognostic stratification for VSA patients [8]. A total of 7 variables, including history of OHCA (4 points), smoking, rest angina alone, organic coronary stenosis, multivessel spasm during the spasm provocation tests (2 points per each), ST-segment elevation during angina, and β-blocker use (1 point per each) were chosen for the JCSA score. Of note, MACE were incrementally documented in line with the low-risk, intermediate-risk, high-risk (2.5%, 7.0% and 13.0%, $P < 0.001$). Among the 3 risk groups, clear prognostic utility of the JCSA scoring system for MACE was confirmed throughout the follow-up period. Thus, JCSA risk score is useful for the treatment and assessment of the risk stratification of future cardiovascular events in VSA patients [8].

4.4   Biomarkers and Cardiac Imaging as a Treatment Efficacy for Coronary Artery Spasm

We previously demonstrated that Rho-kinase activity in circulating neutrophils, determined by the extent of phosphorylation of myosin-binding subunit (MBS, a substrate of Rho-kinase), is significantly enhanced in VSA patients as compared with controls, which is a useful noninvasive diagnostic biomarker to assess the vasospastic disorder and the disease activity [9]. In this study, Rho-kinase activity in circulating neutrophils was expressed as the ratio of phosphorylated MBS (p-MBS) to total MBS (t-MBS). A p-MBS ratio of 1.18 was identified as the best cutoff level to predict the diagnosis of VSA. The Rho-kinase activity was found to show the association with the severity of angina symptoms, and was able to correspond to the significant reduction in the disease activity after medical treatment. When we divided 174 VSA patients into 2 groups by a cutoff value (1.20), VSA patients with higher Rho-kinase activity ($\geq$1.20) had significantly worse prognosis [46]. In this study, a p-MBS ratio of 1.24 was identified as the best cutoff level to predict future cardiac events in VSA patients. Of note, combination of Rho-kinase activity with the JCSA risk score dramatically improved the prognostic impact in VSA patients as compared with either alone [46].

We previously demonstrated that chronic inflammatory changes in the coronary adventitia play roles in the pathogenesis of coronary artery spasm through Rho-kinase activation and resultant vascular smooth muscle hypercontraction [1, 26–28, 40, 41, 47–50]. We thus developed novel imaging approaches for evaluating the extent of coronary adventitial inflammatory changes in VSA patients in vivo. Indeed, we were able to demonstrate that optimal coherence tomography (OCT)-delineated adventitial VV formation was significantly enhanced at the spastic segments of VSA patients as compared with those of the control subjects [51, 52]. Notably, VV formation was significantly increased in the group with high JCSA score than that with the low or intermediate score. We then demonstrated that coronary perivascular adipose tissue (PVAT) volume measured by CT coronary angiography was increased at the spastic segment of VSA patients [53]. In addition, ^{18}F-fluorodeoxyglucose (^{18}F-FDG) positron emission tomographic (PET) imaging allows us to evaluate inflammatory changes of coronary PVAT in pigs in vivo [54]. The extent of PVAT inflammation was expressed as a target to background ratio (TBR), the standardized uptake value (SUV) corrected for blood activity by dividing the average blood SUV estimated from the ascending aorta. Importantly, using this imaging approach with ^{18}F-FDG PET, we demonstrated that coronary PVAT inflammatory changes were more enhanced at the spastic coronary segments of VSA patients as compared with those of controls [55]. Importantly, inflammatory changes measured by ^{18}F-FDG PET were significantly suppressed after medical treatment (Fig. 4.6) and also associated with improvement of angina symptom (Fig. 4.7). Taken together, these biomarkers and imaging approaches provide better understanding of the pathogenesis and treatment efficacy of coronary artery spasm in VSA patients (Fig. 4.8) [55–57].

4.5   Future Perspectives

Although the long-term prognosis of VSA patients is usually good, refractory VSA and major cardiac events, including acute myocardial infarction and sudden cardiac death, remain important issues. Further studies are needed to improve the understanding of this pathophysiology and to develop new effective therapies.

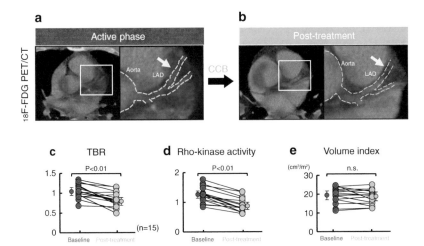

Fig. 4.6 Usefulness of ^{18}F-FDG PET/CT images and assessment of Rho-kinase activity before and after medical treatment in VSA patients(A ~ E). Representative ^{18}F-FDG PET/CT images with a VSA patient at baseline (**a**) and follow-up (**b**). Coronary perivascular FDG uptake was markedly decreased in the spastic LAD after medical treatment. Quantitative analysis showed that coronary perivascular TBR (**c**) and Rho-kinase activity (**d**) were significantly decreased after medical treatment, although coronary perivascular adipose tissue volume index (**e**) was not significantly decreased. ^{18}F-FDG PET/CT = ^{18}F-fluorodeoxyglucose positron emission tomography/computed tomography; CT = computed tomography; FDG = fluorodeoxyglucose; VSA = vasospastic angina. (Reproduced from Ohyama K, et al. [55])

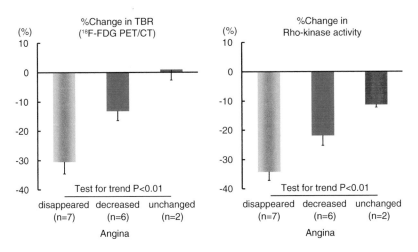

Fig. 4.7 Symptom improvement after medical treatment and changes in coronary perivascular FDG uptake and those in Rho-kinase activity. There were significant trends between the extent of symptom improvement and percent change in coronary perivascular TBR and that of Rho-kinase activity during a median follow-up of 23 months in the group with VSA. FDG = Fluorodeoxyglucose; TBR = target-to-background ratio; VSA = vasospastic angina. (Reproduced from Ohyama K, et al. [55])

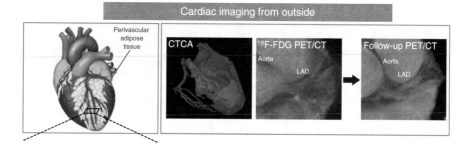

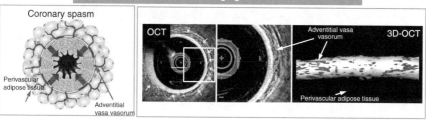

Fig. 4.8 Multimodality Imaging in VSA Patients. Coronary spasm is associated with inflammation of coronary adventitia and PVAT, as evident by ^{18}F-FDG PET/CT and OCT. In addition, ^{18}F-FDG PET/CT could be useful for disease activity assessment. FDG = Fluorodeoxyglucose; PET = positron emission tomography; OCT = optical coherence tomography; VSA = vasospastic angina. (Reproduced from Ohyama K, et al. [55])

Acknowledgement We would like to thank Masahiro Mohri, MD, PhD, Yoshihiro Fukumoto, MD, PhD, Akihiro Masumoto, MD, PhD, Kunio Morishige, MD, Tadashi Kandabashi, MD, PhD, PhD, Junko Hiroki, MD, PhD, Satoshi Yasuda, MD, PhD, Morihiko Takeda MD, PhD, Takashi Shiroto, MD, PhD, Ryuji Tsuburaya, MD, PhD, Kentaro Aizawa, MD, PhD, Yoku Kikuchi, MD, PhD, Yusuke Takagi, MD, PhD, Masayasu Komatsu, MD, PhD, Taro Nihei, MD, PhD, Yuji Odaka, MD, PhD, Tasuku Watanabe, MD, Satoshi Tsuchiya, MD, Jun Sugisawa, MD, and Kohichi Sato, MD, for their contributions to the research works at the Department of Cardiovascular Medicine, Kyushu University Graduate School of Medicine and Tohoku University Graduate School of Medicine.

References

1. Shimokawa H. 2014 Williams Harvey lecture: importance of coronary vasomotion abnormalities-from bench to bedside. Eur Heart J. 2014;35:3180–93. https://doi.org/10.1093/eurheartj/ehu427.
2. Pristipino C, Beltrame JF, Finocchiaro ML, Hattori R, Fujita M, Mongiardo P, Cianflone D, Sanna T, Sasayama S, Maseri A. Major racial differences in coronary constrictor response between Japanese and Caucasians with recent myocardial infarction. Circulation. 2000;101:1102–8. https://doi.org/10.1161/01.CIR.101.10.1102.

3. Beltrame JF, Sasayama S, Maseri A. Racial heterogeneity in coronary artery vasomotor reactivity: differences between Japanese and Caucasian patients. J Am Coll Cardiol. 1999;33:1442–52. https://doi.org/10.1016/s0735-1097(99)00073-x.

4. Ong P, Athanasiadis A, Hill S, Vogelsberg H, Voehringer M, Sechtem U. Coronary artery spasm as a frequent cause of acute coronary syndrome. The CASPAR (Coronary artery spasm in patients with acute coronary syndrome) study. J Am Coll Cardiol. 2008;52:528–30. https://doi.org/10.1016/j.jacc.2008.04.050.

5. Ong P, Athanasiadis A, Borgulya G, Vokshi I, Bastiaenen R, Kubik S, Hill S, Schäufele T, Mahrholdt H, Kaski JC, Sechtem U. Clinical usefulness, angiographic characteristics, and safety evaluation of intracoronary acetylcholine provocation testing among 921 consecutive white patients with unobstructed coronary arteries. Circulation. 2014;129:1723–30. https://doi.org/10.1161/CIRCULATIONAHA.113.004096.

6. Sato K, Takahashi J, Odaka Y, Suda A, Sueda S, Teragawa H, Ishii K, Kiyooka T, Hirayama A, Sumiyoshi T, Tanabe Y, Kimura K, Kaikita K, Ong O, Sechtem U, Camici PG, Kaski JC, Crea F, Beltrame JF, Shimokawa H, Japanese Coronary Spasm Association. Clinical characteristics and long-term prognosis of contemporary patients with vasospastic angina Ethnic differences detected in an international comparative study. Int J Cardiol. 2019;291:13–8. https://doi.org/10.1016/j.ijcard.2019.02.038.

7. JCS joint working group. Guidelines for diagnosis and treatment of patients with vasospastic angina (Coronary spastic angina). Circ J. 2014;78:2779–801. https://doi.org/10.1253/circj.CJ-66-0098.

8. Takagi Y, Takahashi J, Yasuda S, Miyata S, Tsunoda R, Ogata Y, Seki A, Sumiyoshi T, Matsui M, Goto T, Tanabe Y, Sueda S, Sato T, Ogawa S, Kubo N, Momomura S, Ogawa H, Shimokawa H. Prognostic stratification of patients with vasospastic angina: a comprehensive clinical risk score developed by the Japanese Coronary Spasm Association. J Am Coll Cardiol. 2013;62:1144–53. https://doi.org/10.1016/j.jacc.2013.07.018.

9. Kikuchi Y, Yasuda S, Aizawa K, Tsuburaya R, Ito Y, Takeda M, Nakayama M, Ito K, Takahashi J, Shimokawa H. Enhanced Rho-kinase activity in circulating neutrophils of patients with vasospastic angina. A possible biomarker for diagnosis and disease activity assessment. J Am Coll Cardiol. 2011;58:1231–7. https://doi.org/10.1016/j.jacc.2011.05.046.

10. Ohyama K, Matsumoto Y, Takanami K, Ota H, Nishimiya K, Sugisawa J, Tsuchiya S, Amamizu H, Uzuka H, Suda A, Shindo T, Kikuchi Y, Hao K, Tsuburaya R, Takahasi J, Miyata S, Sakata Y, Takase K, Shimokawa H. Coronary adventitial and perivascular adipose tissue inflammation in patients with vasospastic angina. J Am Coll Cardiol. 2018;71:414–25. https://doi.org/10.1016/j.jacc.2017.11.046.

11. Hiroki J, Shimokawa H, Higashi M, Morikawa K, Kandabashi T, Kawamura N, Kubota T, Ichiki T, Amano M, Kaibuchi K, Takeshita A. Inflammatory stimuli upregulate Rho-kinase in human coronary vascular smooth muscle cells. J Mol Cell Cardiol. 2004;37:537–46.

12. Yasue H, Hirai N, Mizuno Y, Harada E, Itoh T, Yoshimura M, Kugiyama K, Ogawa H. Low-grade inflammation, thrombogenicity, and atherogenic lipid profile in cigarette smokers. Circ J. 2006;70:8–13. https://doi.org/10.1253/circj.70.8.

13. Miwa K, Fujita M, Miyagi Y. Beneficial effects of smoking cessation on the short-term prognosis for variant angina--validation of the smoking status by urinary cotinine measurements. Int J Cardiol. 1994;44:151–6. https://doi.org/10.1016/0167-5273(94)90019-1.

14. Yeung AC, Vekshtein VI, Krantz DS, Vita JA, Ryan TJ Jr, Ganz P, Selwyn AP. The effect of atherosclerosis on the vasomotor response of coronary arteries to mental stress. N Engl J Med. 1991;325:1551–6. https://doi.org/10.1056/NEJM199111283252205.

15. Oda H, Suzuki M, Oniki T, Kishi Y, Numano F. Alcohol and coronary spasm. Angiology. 1994;45:187–97. https://doi.org/10.1177/000331979404500303.

16. Kalsner S. Cocaine sensitization of coronary artery contractions: mechanism of drug-induced spasm. J Pharmacol Exp Ther. 1993;264:1132–40.

17. Hizume T, Morikawa K, Takaki A, Abe K, Sunagawa K, Amano M, Kaibuchi K, Kubo C, Shimokawa H. Sustained elevation of serum cortisol level causes sensitization of coronary

vasoconstricting responses in pigs in vivo. A possible link between stress and coronary vaso-spasm. Circ Res. 2006;99:767–75. https://doi.org/10.1161/01.RES.0000244093.69985.2f.

18. Yasue H, Takizawa A, Nagao M, Nishida S, Horie M, Kubota J, Omote S, Takaoka K, Okumura K. Long-term prognosis for patients with variant angina and influential factors. Circulation. 1988;78:1–9. https://doi.org/10.1161/01.cir.78.1.1.

19. Crea F, Merz CNB, Beltrame JF, Berry C, Camici PG, Kaski JC, Ong P, Pepine CJ, Sechtem U. Mechanisms and diagnostic evaluation of persistent or recurrent angina following percutaneous coronary revascularization. Eur Heart J. 2019;40:2455–62. https://doi.org/10.1093/eurheartj/ehy857.

20. Shiroto T, Yasuda S, Tsuburaya R, Ito Y, Takahashi J, Ito K, Ishibashi-Ueda H, Shimokawa H. Role of Rho-kinase in the pathogenesis of coronary hyperconstricting responses induced by drug-eluting stents in pigs in vivo. J Am Coll Cardiol. 2009;54:2321–9. https://doi.org/10.1016/j.jacc.2009.07.045.

21. Tsuburaya R, Takahashi J, Nakamura A, Nozaki E, Sugi M, Yamamoto Y, Hiramoto T, Horiguchi S, Inoue K, Goto T, Kato A, Shinozaki T, Ishida E, Miyata S, Yasuda S, Shimokawa H. Beneficial effects of long-acting nifedipine on coronary vasomotion abnormalities after drug-eluting stent implantation: The NOVEL study. Eur Heart J. 2016;37:2713–21. https://doi.org/10.1093/eurheartj/ehw256.

22. Fukumoto Y, Yasuda S, Ito A, Shimokawa H. Prognostic effects of benidipine in patients with vasospastic angina: comparison with diltiazem and amlodipine. J Cardiovasc Pharmacol. 2008;51:253–7. https://doi.org/10.1097/FJC.0b013e3181624b05.

23. Nishigaki K, Inoue Y, Yamanouchi Y, Fukumoto Y, Yasuda S, Sueda S, Urata H, Shimokawa H, Minatoguchi S. Prognostic effects of calcium channel blockers in patients with vasospastic angina—a meta-analysis. Circ J. 2010;74:1943–50. https://doi.org/10.1253/circj.CJ-10-0292.

24. Takahashi J, Nihei T, Takagi Y, Miyata S, Odaka Y, Tsunoda R, Seki A, Sumiyoshi T, Matsui M, Goto T, Tanabe Y, Sueda S, Momomura S, Yasuda S, Ogawa H, Shimokawa H, Japanese Coronary Spasm Association. Prognostic impact of chronic nitrate therapy in patients with vasospastic angina: multicentre registry study of the Japanese coronary spasm association. Eur Heart J. 2015;36:228–37. https://doi.org/10.1093/eurheartj/ehu313.

25. Katsumata N, Shimokawa H, Seto M, Kozai T, Yamawaki T, Kuwata K, Egashira K, Ikegaki I, Asano T, Sasaki Y, Takeshita A. Enhanced myosin light chain phosphorylations as a central mechanism for coronary artery spasm in a swine model with interleukin-1β. Circulation. 1997;96:4357–63. https://doi.org/10.1161/01.cir.96.12.4357.

26. Shimokawa H, Seto M, Katsumata N, Amano M, Kozai T, Yamawaki T, Kuwata K, Kandabashi T, Egashira K, Ikegaki I, Asano T, Kaibuchi K, Takeshita A. Rho-kinase-mediated pathway induces enhanced myosin light chain phosphorylations in a swine model of coronary artery spasm. Cardiovasc Res. 1999;43:1138–41. https://doi.org/10.1016/s0008-6363(99)00144-3.

27. Shimokawa H, Ito A, Fukumoto Y, Kadokami T, Nakaike R, Sakata M, Takayanagi T, Egashira K, Takeshita A. Chronic treatment with interleukin-1β induces coronary intimal lesions and vasospastic responses in pigs in vivo: the role of platelet-derived growth factor. J Clin Invest. 1996;97:769–76. https://doi.org/10.1172/JCI118476.

28. Kandabashi T, Shimokawa H, Miyata K, Kunihiro I, Kawano Y, Fukata Y, Higo T, Egashira K, Takahashi S, Kaibuchi K, Takeshita A. Inhibition of myosin phosphatase by upregulated Rho-kinase plays a key role for coronary artery spasm in a porcine model with interleukin-1beta. Circulation. 2000;10:1319–23. https://doi.org/10.1161/01.CIR.101.11.1319.

29. Kandabashi T, Shimokawa H, Mukai Y, Matoba T, Kunihiro I, Morikawa K, Ito M, Takahashi S, Kaibuchi K, Takeshita A. Involvement of Rho-kinase in agonists-induced contractions of arteriosclerotic human arteries. Arterioscler Thromb Vasc Biol. 2002;22:243–8. https://doi.org/10.1161/hq0202.104274.

30. Masumoto A, Mohri M, Shimokawa H, Urakami L, Usui M, Takeshita A. Suppression of coronary artery spasm by the Rho-kinase inhibitor fasudil in patients with vasospastic angina. Circulation. 2002;105:1545–7. https://doi.org/10.1161/hc1002.105938.

31. Fischell TA, McDonald TV, Grattan MT, Miller DC, Stadius ML. Occlusive coronary-artery spasm as a cause of acute myocardial infarction after coronary-artery bypass grafting. N Engl J Med. 1989;320:400–1. https://doi.org/10.1056/NEJM198902093200617.

32. Inokuchi K, Ito A, Fukumoto Y, Matoba T, Shiose A, Nishida T, Masuda M, Morita S, Shimokawa H. Usefulness of fasudil, a Rho-kinase inhibitor, to treat intractable severe coronary spasm after coronary artery bypass surgery. J Cardiovasc Pharmacol. 2004;44:275–7. https://doi.org/10.1097/01.fjc.0000134775.76636.3f.

33. Shimokawa H, Hiramori K, Iinuma H, Hosoda S, Kishida H, Osada H, Katagiri T, Yamauchi K, Yui Y, Minamino T, Nakashima M, Kato K. Anti-anginal effect of fasudil, a Rho-kinase inhibitor, in patients with stable effort angina: a multicenter study. J Cardiovasc Pharmacol. 2002;40:751–61. https://doi.org/10.1097/00005344-200211000-00013.

34. Sueda S, Miyoshi T, Sasaki Y, Sakaue T, Habara H, Kohno H. Approximately half of patients with coronary spastic angina had pathologic exercise tests. J Cardiol. 2016;68:13–9. https://doi.org/10.1016/j.jjcc.2016.01.009.

35. Takeda M, Shiba N, Takahashi J, Shimokawa H. A case report of very late stent thrombosis with peri-stent coronary artery aneurysm and stent-related coronary vasospasm. Cardiovasc Interv Ther. 2013;28:272–8. https://doi.org/10.1007/s12928-012-0155-7.

36. Aizawa K, Yasuda S, Takahashi J, Takii T, Kikuchi Y, Tsuburaya R, Ito Y, Ito K, Nakayama M, Takeda M, Shimokawa H. Involvement of Rho-kinase activation in the pathogenesis of coronary hyperconstricting responses induced by drug-eluting stents in patients with coronary artery disease. Circ J. 2012;76:2552–60. https://doi.org/10.1253/circj.CJ-12-0662.

37. Yasue H, Mizuno Y, Harada E, Itoh T, Nakagawa H, Nakayama M, Ogawa H, Tayama S, Honda T, Hokimoto S, Ohshima S, Hokamura Y, Kugiyama K, Horie M, Yoshimura M, Harada M, Uemura S, Saito Y, SCAST (Statin and Coronary Artery Spasm Trial) Investigators. Effects of a 3-hydroxy-3-methylglutaryl coenzyme A reductase inhibitor, fluvastatin, on coronary spasm after withdrawal of calcium-channel blockers. J Am Coll Cardiol. 2008;51:1742–8. https://doi.org/10.1016/j.jacc.2007.12.049.

38. Satake K, Lee JD, Shimizu H, Ueda T, Nakamura T. Relation between severity of magnesium deficiency and frequency of anginal attacks in men with variant angina. J Am Coll Cardiol. 1996;28:897–902. https://doi.org/10.1016/s0735-1097(96)00256-2.

39. Teragawa H, Kato M, Yamagata T, Matsuura H, Kajiyama G. The preventive effect of magnesium on coronary spasm in patients with vasospastic angina. Chest. 2000;118:1690–5. https://doi.org/10.1378/chest.118.6.1690.

40. Uzuka H, Matsumoto Y, Nishimiya K, Ohyama K, Suzuki H, Amamizu H, Morosawa S, Hirano M, Shindo T, Kikuchi Y, Hao K, Shiroto T, Ito K, Takahashi J, Fukuda K, Miyata S, Funaki Y, Ishibashi-Ueda H, Yasuda S, Shimokawa H. Renal denervation suppresses coronary hyperconstricting responses after drug-eluting stent implantation in pigs in vivo through the kidney-brain-heart axis. Arterioscler Thromb Vasc Biol. 2017;37:1869–80. https://doi.org/10.1161/ATVBAHA.117.309777.

41. Nishimiya K, Matsumoto Y, Uzuka H, Ogata T, Hirano M, Shindo T, Hasebe Y, Tsuburaya R, Shiroto T, Takahashi J, Ito K, Shimokawa H. Beneficial effects of a novel bioabsorbable polymer coating on enhanced coronary vasoconstricting responses after drug-eluting stent implantation in pigs in vivo. J Am Coll Cardiol Caardiovasc Interv. 2016;9:281–91. https://doi.org/10.1016/j.jcin.2015.09.041.

42. Sugisawa J, Matsumoto Y, Suda A, Tsuchiya S, Ohyama K, Takeuchi M, Nishimiya K, Akizuki M, Sato K, Kajitani S, Ota H, Ikeda S, Shindo T, Kikuchi Y, Hao K, Shiroto T, Takahashi J, Miyata S, Sakata Y, Takase K, Kohzuki M, Shimokawa H. Exercise training ameliorates vasodilator capacity of coronary microvessels in patients with vasospastic angina -a new therapeutic approach for the coronary functional disorder. Circulation. 2019;140:Abstract 12707.

43. Watanabe T, Matsumoto Y, Amamizu H, Morosawa S, Ohyama K, Sugisawa J, Tsuchiya S, Sato K, Suda A, Shindo T, Ikeda S, Nishimiya K, Kikuchi Y, Hao K, Shiroto T, Takahashi J, Shimokawa H. Low-intensity pulsed ultrasound ameliorates DES-induced coronary adven-

titial inflammation and hyperconstricting responses in pigs in vivo - A novel non-invasive therapy for coronary inflammation. Eur Heart J. 2019;40:Supplement_1, ehz748.0144. https://doi.org/10.1093/eurheartj/ehz748.0144.

44. Komatsu M, Takahashi J, Fukuda K, Takagi Y, Shiroto T, Nakano M, Kondo M, Tsuburaya R, Hao K, Nishimiya K, Nihei T, Matsumoto Y, Ito K, Sakata Y, Miyata S, Shimokawa H. Usefulness of testing for coronary artery spasm and programmed ventricular stimulation in survivors of out-of-hospital cardiac arrest. Circ Arrhythm Electrophysiol. 2016;9:e003798. https://doi.org/10.1161/CIRCEP.115.003798.

45. Ahn JM, Lee KH, Yoo SY, Cho YR, Suh J, Shin ES, Lee JH, Shin DI, Kim SH, Baek SH, Seung KB, Nam CW, Jin ES, Lee SW, Oh JH, Jang JH, Park HW, Yoon NS, Cho JG, Lee CH, Park DW, Kang SJ, Lee SW, Kim J, Kim YH, Nam KB, Lee CW, Choi KJ, Song JK, Kim YH, Park SW, Park SJ. Prognosis of variant angina manifesting as aborted sudden cardiac death. J Am Coll Cardiol. 2016;68:137–45. https://doi.org/10.1016/j.jacc.2016.04.050.

46. Nihei T, Takahashi J, Hao K, Kikuchi Y, Odaka Y, Tsuburaya R, Nishimiya K, Matsumoto Y, Ito K, Miyata S, Sakata Y, Shimokawa H. Prognostic impacts of Rho-kinase activity in circulating leukocytes in patients with vasospastic angina. Eur Heart J. 2018;39:952–9. https://doi.org/10.1093/eurheartj/ehx657.

47. Amamizu H, Matsumoto Y, Morosawa S, Ohyama K, Uzuka H, Hirano M, Nishimiya K, Gokon Y, Watanabe-Asaka T, Hayashi M, Miyata S, Kamei T, Kawai Y, Shimokawa H. Cardiac lymphatic dysfunction causes drug-eluting stent-induced coronary hyperconstricting responses in pigs in vivo. Arterioscler Thromb Vasc Biol. 2019;39:741–53. https://doi.org/10.1161/ATVBAHA.119.312396.

48. Nishimiya K, Matsumoto Y, Shindo T, Hanawa K, Hasebe Y, Tsuburaya R, Shiroto T, Takahashi J, Ito K, Ishibashi-Ueda H, Yasuda S, Shimokawa H. Association of adventitial vasa vasorum and inflammation with coronary hyperconstriction after drug-eluting stent implantation in pigs in vivo. Circ J. 2015;79:1787–98. https://doi.org/10.1253/circj.CJ-15-0149.

49. Nishimiya K, Matsumoto Y, Takahashi J, Uzuka H, Odaka Y, Nihei T, Hao K, Tsuburaya R, Ito K, Shimokawa H. In vivo visualization of adventitial vasa vasorum of the human coronary artery on optical frequency domain imaging. Validation study. Circ J. 2014;78:2516–8. https://doi.org/10.1253/circj.cj-14-0485.

50. Nishimiya K, Matsumoto Y, Uzuka H, Oyama K, Tanaka A, Taruya A, Ogata T, Hirano M, Shindo T, Hanawa K, Hasebe Y, Hao K, Tsuburaya R, Takahashi J, Miyata S, Ito K, Akasaka T, Shimokawa H. Accuracy of optical frequency domain imaging for evaluation of coronary adventitial vasa vasorum formation after stent implantation in pigs and humans. A validation study. Circ J. 2015;79:1323–31. https://doi.org/10.1253/circj.CJ-15-0078.

51. Nishimiya K, Matsumoto Y, Uzuka H, Ohyama K, Hao K, Tsuburaya R, Shiroto T, Takahashi J, Ito K, Shimokawa H. Focal vasa vasorum formation in patients with focal coronary vasospasm. -An optical frequency domain imaging study. Circ J. 2016;80:2252–4.

52. Nishimiya K, Matsumoto Y, Takahashi J, Uzuka H, Wang H, Tsuburaya R, Hao K, Ohyama K, Odaka Y, Miyata S, Ito K, Shimokawa H. Enhanced adventitial vasa vasorum formation in patients with vasospastic angina. J Am Coll Cardiol. 2016;67:598–600. https://doi.org/10.1016/j.jacc.2015.11.031.

53. Ohyama K, Matsumoto Y, Nishimiya K, Hao K, Tsuburaya R, Ota H, Amamizu H, Uzuka H, Takahashi J, Ito K, Shimokawa H. Increased coronary perivascular adipose tissue volume in patients with vasospastic angina. Circ J. 2016;80:1653–6. https://doi.org/10.1253/circj.CJ-16-0213.

54. Ohyama K, Matsumoto Y, Amamizu H, Uzuka H, Nishimiya K, Morosawa S, Hirano M, Watabe H, Funaki Y, Miyata S, Takahashi J, Ito K, Shimokawa H. Association of coronary perivascular adipose tissue inflammation and DES-induced coronary hyperconstriction responses in pigs. -^{18}F-FDG PET imaging study. Arterior Thromb Vasc Biol. 2017;37:1757–64. https://doi.org/10.1161/ATVBAHA.117.309843.

55. Ohyama K, Matsumoto Y, Takanami K, Ota H, Nishimiya K, Sugisawa J, Tsuchiya S, Amamizu H, Uzuka H, Suda A, Shindo T, Kikuchi Y, Hao K, Tsuburaya R, Takahashi J, Miyata S, Sakata Y, Takase K, Shimokawa H. Coronary adventitial and perivascular adipose tissue inflam-

mation in patients with vasospastic angina. J Am Coll Cardiol. 2018;71:414–25. https://doi.org/10.1016/j.jacc.2017.11.046.

56. Ohyama K, Matsumoto M, Shimokawa H. Coronary artery spasm and perivascular adipose tissue inflammation: insights from translational imaging research. Eur Cardiol. 2019;14:6–9. https://doi.org/10.15420/ecr.2019.3.2.

57. Nishimiya K, Matsumoto Y, Shimokawa H. Viewpoint: Recent advances in intracoronary imaging for vasa vasorum visualisation. Eur Cardio Rev. 2017;12:121–3. https://doi.org/10.15420/ecr.2017:13:1.

Part II
Coronary Microvascular Dysfunction

Chapter 5
Epidemiology of Coronary Microvascular Dysfunction

Peter Ong and Hiroaki Shimokawa

Abstract Coronary microvascular dysfunction (CMD) is a frequent clinical condition leading to angina pectoris and/or shortness of breath in various forms of cardiovascular disease. Several invasive and non-invasive assessments are available for a comprehensive evaluation of the underlying microvascular abnormalities (e.g. coronary flow velocity reserve (CFR) via transthoracic Doppler echocardiography, cardiac magnetic resonance imaging or positron emission tomography, invasive assessment of CFR and microvascular resistance using adenosine as well as the assessment of microvascular coronary spasm using acetylcholine). It is consensus that impaired microvascular vasodilatory function, but also enhanced microvascular vasoconstriction/spasm represent important mechanisms for CMD. The clinical presentation as well as the methods applied for investigation of CMD is associated with the prevalence of CMD. Overall, in patients with signs and symptoms of myocardial ischemia yet unobstructed coronary arteries, CMD can be found in approximately 50–60% of cases. However, the epidemiology of CMD is still difficult to assess. Novel diagnostic techniques involving smartphone-based ECG recordings offer a direct assessment of ischemic ECG shifts during a chest pain attack. The broad applicability of this technology may also influence the epidemiology of CMD. This chapter reviews the available epidemiological data on CMD in patients with angina and unobstructed coronary arteries.

Keywords Coronary microvascular dysfunction · Epidemiology · Prevalence · Acetylcholine · Coronary flow reserve

P. Ong
Department of Cardiology, Robert-Bosch-Krankenhaus, Stuttgart, Germany
e-mail: Peter.Ong@rbk.de

H. Shimokawa (✉)
Department of Cardiovascular Medicine, Tohoku University Graduate School of Medicine, Sendai, Miyagi, Japan
e-mail: shimo@cardio.med.tohoku.ac.jp

Abbreviations

ACh	Acetylcholine
ACS	Acute coronary syndrome
APV	Average peak velocity
CAD	Coronary artery disease
CFR	Coronary flow reserve
CMD	Coronary microvascular dysfunction
CSX	Cardiac syndrome X
CTCA	Computed tomography coronary angiography
ECG	Electrocardiogram
FFR	Fractional flow reserve
IDP	Interventional diagnostic procedure
LCA	Left coronary artery
MINOCA	Myocardial infarction with non-obstructive coronary arteries
NOCAD	Non-obstructive coronary artery disease
NSTEMI	Non-ST-elevation myocardial infarction
PET	Positron emission tomography
RCA	Right coronary artery
STEMI	ST-elevation myocardial infarction

5.1 Introduction

Coronary microcirculation plays a pivotal role in coronary blood flow regulation in various forms of cardiovascular disease [1]. Commonly, microvessels are defined as vessels with a diameter of <500 μm. Remodelling of the coronary microcirculation in response to various stimuli may result in structural and functional alterations [2]. Various clinical conditions, such as hypertension, diabetes, hypercholesterolemia, smoking, obesity and others, have been shown to adversely affect the coronary microcirculation [3]. Clinically, coronary microvascular dysfunction (CMD) can be associated with epicardial atherosclerotic disease, myocardial disease, iatrogenic causes and in the absence of the latter conditions. This allows classification into four different groups as suggested by Crea and Camici [1]. Diagnosing CMD in patients without myocardial or epicardial coronary disease represents a special challenge for the clinical cardiologist. Studies have shown that the prevalence of CMD in patients with unobstructed coronary arteries is high and that their prognosis is not benign. Thus, assessment of the integrity of the coronary microcirculation is important because of its prognostic impact [4]. Depending on the clinical presentation of the patient and the co-existing comorbidities, the clinical cardiologist has to decide which assessments (non-invasive and/or

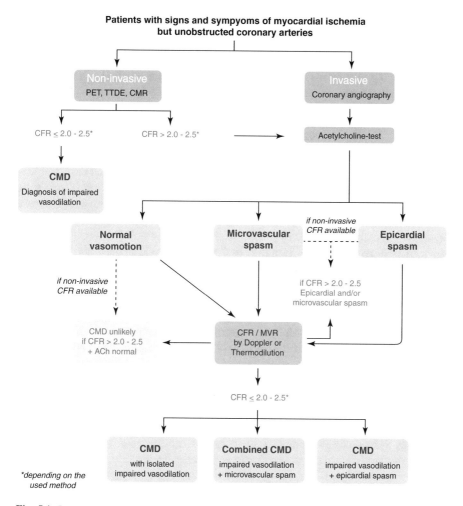

Fig. 5.1 Interventional diagnostic procedure (IDP), proposed by Ong et al. [5], including both non-invasive and invasive techniques in symptomatic patients with unobstructed coronary arteries and suspected CMD. *CFR* coronary flow reserve, *CMR* cardiovascular magnetic resonance, *MVR* microvascular resistance, *PET* positron emission tomography, *TTDE* transthoracic Doppler echocardiography. (Reproduced from Ong et al. [5])

invasive) are appropriate. A proposed diagnostic workup including both non-invasive and invasive techniques is shown in Fig. 5.1. Depending on the diagnostic methods applied for the investigation of CMD, there is a variation in the prevalence of CMD. This chapter gives a contemporary overview of the epidemiology of CMD in patients with signs and symptoms of myocardial ischemia yet unobstructed coronary arteries.

5.2 Historical Background

Long before the discovery of coronary angiography and the advent of invasive cardiology, physicians all over the world have treated patients with chest pain. In the absence of any detailed information about structural or functional heart disease, they could only speculate about the origin of the patient's symptoms. However, the description of the patient's symptoms was one of the most important tasks in which many of these physicians were masters. One of them was William Heberden, a British physician who lived from 1710 until 1801. He was one of the first physicians to describe chest pain as "angina pectoris" a term that has survived until today. Traditionally, the term "angina" arose from about two centuries before his time and was used to describe throat pain, accompanied by a feeling of anxiety. In Heberden's description, angina pectoris was a thoracic discomfort, frequently retrosternal pain, with radiation to the left arm. The symptoms usually occurred during exertion and subsided at rest [6].

With the discovery of the ECG in 1903 by Eindhoven, physicians were able to correlate chest pain symptoms with ischemic ECG changes. Based on the initial description by Heberden [6], it was found that patients with exertional chest pain frequently showed ischemic ECG changes during exercise leading to the term "typical angina". In contrast, others made the observation that patients with resting chest pain could have transient ST-segment elevation on the 12-lead ECG while their exercise capacity was preserved which led to the term "variant angina" by Prinzmetal in 1959 [7]. Prinzmetal assumed that this phenomenon was based on transient spasms of the coronary arteries, and only later it was found out that a substantial proportion of his patients suffered from additional stenosing epicardial disease on autopsy. The description of patients with variant angina and unobstructed coronary arteries was made shortly after and termed "variant of the variant". Although this only fostered the confusion of terminology in this area of cardiology, it should be acknowledged that with the advent of coronary angiography it became apparent that many patients with angina pectoris had unobstructed coronary arteries. In an early study by Proudfit in 1978, it was documented that the prognosis of patients with angina pectoris correlated with the severity of their symptoms, the arteries affected and with an impaired left ventricular function [8]. Moreover, it was previously shown in 1966 that 37% of all patients had unobstructed coronary arteries (<30% luminal obstruction) [9]. Comprehensive research was carried out and Arbogast and Bourassa showed that rapid pacing paradoxically resulted in enhanced left ventricular function in patients with angina but normal coronary arteries, called "group X" [10]. This phenomenon led to the introduction of the term "syndrome X", a label that was commonly used to describe these patients at the time (i.e. chest pain and unobstructed coronary arteries). In 1988, Cannon and Epstein showed that a substantial percentage of patients with angina and unobstructed coronaries exhibited a coronary microvascular disorder and thus introduced the term "microvascular angina" [11]. Subsequently, the concept of coronary microvascular spasm was introduced by Mohri et al. suggesting that an increased vasoconstrictive potential of the coronary microvascular system may be another form of microvascular dysfunction [12].

Despite these seminal studies, the focus of research in clinical cardiology shifted towards epicardial coronary artery disease (CAD) with the introduction of percutaneous coronary interventions in the 1980s by Puel and Sigwart [13]. Thus, the pivotal role of the microcirculation in regulating myocardial perfusion [14] and its clinical importance in patients with angina and unobstructed coronary arteries received less attention. In recent times, the topic has gained more and more attention. This is due to an important review article in the *New England Journal of Medicine* in 2007 [1], the improvement of diagnostic assessments and therapeutic pathways in these patients [15, 16] and the body of evidence confirming an unfavourable prognosis in various cohorts of patients with CMD [4, 17].

5.3 Epidemiological Considerations

Epidemiology is defined as "the study and analysis of the distribution (who, when and where), patterns and determinants of health and disease conditions in defined populations" [18] with two important measures, incidence and prevalence. Whereas incidence refers to the frequency of events correlating with time and does thus reflect morbidity in a population [19], prevalence is a measure for the frequency of a disease, by defining a specific part of a defined population at a time that carries either a certain disease or a risk factor [20]. The epidemiology of CMD is difficult to assess as it can be present in various forms of cardiovascular disease. This chapter will focus on the epidemiology of patients with type 1 CMD according to Crea and Camici (i.e. CMD in the absence of coronary and myocardial disease) [1]. Moreover, there are several different tools available to assess CMD, each with a different definition and yield of establishing the diagnosis. On average, the prevalence of CMD in observational studies in patients with NOCAD ranges from 22% to 63% (Table 5.1) [2].

Table 5.1 Prevalence of CMD in observational studies with various testing modalities

Author	Number of patients (n)	Diagnostic approach	Prevalence of CMD %()	Ref.
Cassar et al.	376	Coronary reactivity testing	63	[21]
Hasdai et al.	203	Coronary reactivity testing	59	[22]
Murthy et al.	1218	PET (CFR < 2.0)	53	[4]
Mygind et al.	919	TTDE (CFR < 2.0)	26	[23]
Reis et al.	159	Coronary reactivity testing	47	[24]
Sade et al.	68	TTDE (CFR < 2.0)	40	[25]
Sara et al.	1439	Coronary reactivity testing	64	[26]
Sicari et al.	394	TTDE (CFR < 2.0)	22	[27]
Wei et al.	293	Coronary reactivity testing	49	[28]

A comprehensive analysis of the prevalence of CMD, reported by multiple studies using various testing approaches, revealed an overall prevalence ranging from 22% to 63%

In addition, various taxonomic definitions and descriptions for CMD have been used inconsistently in the literature complicating this aspect even more. A meta-analysis looking at 57 studies in patients with chest pain and unobstructed coronary arteries previously labelled as cardiac syndrome X revealed very heterogeneous inclusion and exclusion criteria. The authors found as many as 9 inclusion and 43 exclusion criteria limiting the comparability of the studies. Moreover, these different criteria had an impact on the estimated incidence of the disease over 1 year treated in a general hospital ranging from 3% to 11%. Interestingly, the meta-analysis revealed a pooled proportion of females of 0.56 (n = 1934 patients, with 95% confidence interval: 0.54–0.59) (Fig. 5.2) [29].

5.4 Definition of Unobstructed Coronary Arteries

Patients with angina and unobstructed coronary arteries are frequently encountered in daily clinical practice. However, the interpretation of epicardial disease regarding its severity has many pitfalls. As previously shown by Bertrand et al., visual assessments of epicardial stenoses by experienced cardiologist are somewhat inaccurate compared to computerized assessments [30]. The authors demonstrated that the degree of epicardial stenosis pre-PCI differed between the cardiologists and the computerized quantitative analysis (80.6 ± 9.7 vs. 73.4 ± 11.1). Interestingly, the assessment after PCI was 18.8% ± 12.3 by the cardiologists and 37.4 ± 14 by the computer system [30]. Moreover, there is no international consensus regarding the definition of unobstructed coronary arteries. A frequently applied criterion is a <50% stenosis based on visual assessment. However, other studies have applied a 30% criterion or even a 70% criterion [9]. With the introduction of invasively available pressure-wire measurements for assessment of hemodynamic relevance of epicardial stenoses, it is recommended to refrain from a percental classification of epicardial stenoses. It is rather advisable to perform pressure-wire assessments of any intermediate epicardial lesion as even epicardial lesions with a 30% stenosis may be hemodynamically relevant as shown by Toth et al. [31]. Thus, contemporary study protocols for the evaluation of CMD should include such pressure-wire measurements in order to not overlook any relevant epicardial stenosis amenable for coronary revascularization.

The improvement of the CTCA technology and its broader applicability has led to several large studies, showing that an initial CTCA approach in patients with suspected CAD is feasible [32]. However, such an approach is limited by the fact that CTCA only delivers information about coronary anatomy but neither on any functional coronary disorders nor on the hemodynamic relevance of any intermediate epicardial lesion. These limitations can be overcome by the CT-FFR technique, where not only anatomic information about epicardial stenoses but also functional information about the hemodynamic relevance of a given lesion is assessed [33, 34]. In addition, a combined assessment of not only CTCA and CT-FFR but also CT-perfusion has been shown to be feasible in clinical studies [35]. The

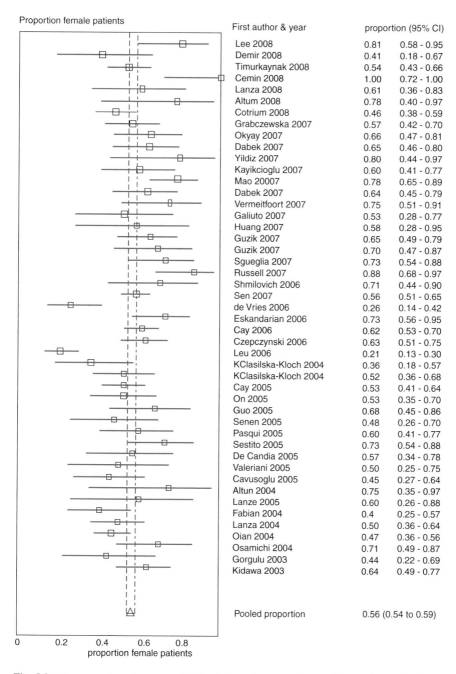

Fig. 5.2 The proportion of women of individual studies regarding cardiac syndrome X (CSD), including 95% confidence intervals. A considerable variation in 47 studies regarding the proportion of women with CSX could be seen with values ranging from 0.21 to 1.0 and a pooled estimate of 0.56 (95% confidence interval: 0.54–0.59). Thus, women suffer significantly more often from CSX compared to men. (Reproduced from Vermeltfoort et al. [29])

development of such imaging techniques represents an attractive and innovative approach for future assessments of such patients in whom a "one stop shop" may be able to provide information about epicardial plaques/stenoses (CTCA), hemodynamic relevance (CT-FFR) as well as impairment of the coronary microcirculation (CT-Perfusion-CFR).

5.5 Prevalence of CMD Depends on Diagnostic Assessments Used

The fact that the coronary microvasculature cannot be visualized in vivo patients makes its assessment a true challenge. Over the past years, multiple non-invasive and invasive methods have been established for the assessment of CMD and their specific use depends not only on the clinical state of the patient, but also on local availability, expertise and cost as well. Non-invasive methods to evaluate the coronary microvasculature include the assessment of coronary flow velocity reserve (CFVR) via transthoracic Doppler echocardiography, cardiac magnetic resonance imaging or positron emission tomography. Invasive methods, on the other hand, comprise the assessment of CFR and microvascular resistance using adenosine as well as the assessment of microvascular coronary spasm using acetylcholine (ACh). The COVADIS (Coronary Vasomotion Disorders International Study) Group has assembled the diagnostic criteria for CMD as shown in Table 5.2 [36]. It has been acknowledged that impaired microvascular vasodilatation as well as enhanced microvascular vasoconstriction/spasm represent mechanisms for microvascular dysfunction. Recently, a new innovative approach titled "interventional diagnostic procedure" (IDP), which allows the invasive assessment of coronary vasoconstrictor and vasodilator abnormalities in combination, has been established (Fig. 5.1) [5].

5.6 Prevalence of Chest Pain and Unobstructed Coronary Arteries and Prevalence of CMD in Acute Coronary Syndrome

Early studies have shown that a substantial proportion of patients with acute coronary syndrome have unobstructed coronary arteries [37]. Hochman et al. showed that ~30% of women and ~14% of men with ACS had no culprit lesion [37]. The frequency of NOCAD was greater in patients with unstable angina compared to those with STEMI or NSTEMI. A more recent meta-analysis of 27 large studies involving a total of 176,502 patients with myocardial infarction showed frequencies of ACS patients without culprit lesion ranging from 1% to 14% (overall prevalence 6%) [38]. Furthermore, patients with ACS and non-obstructive coronary arteries are more likely to be younger, female and it could be observed that they were less likely

Table 5.2 Clinical criteria for suspecting coronary microvascular dysfunction

1.	Symptoms of myocardial ischemia
	(a) Effort and/or rest angina
	(b) Angina equivalents (i.e. shortness of breath)
2.	Absence of obstructive CAD (<50% diameter reduction or FFR > 0.80) by
	(a) Coronary CTA
	(b) Invasive coronary angiography
3.	Objective evidence of myocardial ischemia
	(a) Ischemic ECG changes during an episode of chest pain
	(b) Stress-induced chest pain and/or ischemic ECG changes in the presence or absence of transient/reversible abnormal myocardial perfusion and/or wall motion abnormality
4.	Evidence of impaired coronary microvascular function
	(a) Impaired coronary flow reserve (cut-off values depending on methodology use between ≤ 2.0 and ≤ 2.5)
	(b) Coronary microvascular spasm, defined as reproduction of symptoms, ischemic ECG shills but no epicardial spasm during acetylcholine testing
	(c) Abnormal coronary microvascular resistance indices (e.g. IMR > 25)
	(d) Coronary slow flow phenomenon, defined as TIMI frame count >25

The following criteria should lead to the suspicion of CMD

ECG electrocardiogram, *CAD* coronary artery disease, *CTA* computed tomographic angiography, *FFR* fractional flow reserve, *IMR* index of microcirculatory resistance, *TIMI* thrombolysis in myocardial infarction. (Reproduced from Ong et al. [36])

to have hyperlipidemia compared to those with myocardial infarction and obstructive CAD. Nowadays such patients should be labelled with a working diagnosis of MINOCA (myocardial infarction with non-obstructive coronary arteries) and possible ischemic causes in the setting of ACS without culprit lesion should be investigated according to the so-called "traffic light approach" [39]. This should also involve assessments for CMD. The feasibility to determine a diagnosis of CMD in an ACS setting has been described using non-invasive as well as invasive techniques. A study by Safdar et al. using PET-CFR (cut-off CFR > 2.0 for rate-pressure product corrected values and CFR < 2.5 for uncorrected values) in 195 emergency room patients showed that in nearly half of the patients with chest pain and without MI or CAD, CMD could be diagnosed [40]. A great amount of these patients were females and obese, highlighting the important role of cardiovascular risk factors [40]. Other studies reported the usefulness of investigations for CMD in ACS patients undergoing invasive angiography. Sato et al. [41] showed that ACS patients without culprit lesion may also suffer from microvascular spasm on ACh testing, a finding that was predominantly seen in female patients. In addition, Pirozzolo et al. showed that coronary microvascular spasm, a subtype of CMD, can be frequently found in patients with MINOCA. Indeed, while epicardial spasm could be induced with ACh in 27% of the 96 patients, coronary microvascular spasm was seen in 31% [42]. Furthermore, the prevalence of epicardial spasm could be associated with smoking, a finding, which has been previously described [41].

5.7   Chronic Coronary Syndrome

From the beginning of coronary angiography, patients with angina and unobstructed coronary arteries were not infrequently encountered. Until today, they represent one of the most challenging groups of patients in clinical cardiology. The study by Proudfit et al. in 1966 revealed that 37% of 1000 patients undergoing coronary angiography had unobstructed coronary arteries (<30% diameter obstruction) [9]. Such numbers were confirmed in several large registry studies. In more recent times, a seminal publication from the USA by Patel et al. revealed that more than 50% of patients with suspected CAD had NOCAD [43]. This led to speculations as to whether or not the inclusion criteria and the indication for invasive angiography should be optimized. Moreover, these findings also fostered prospective studies for the investigation of coronary vasomotor disorders as an explanation for the patient's symptoms in this setting [44]. A study by Jespersen et al. confirmed previous observations that a diagnosis of NOCAD is not benign with an event rate of 1.7%/year [45]. Frequently, cardiovascular risk factors lead to the pathophysiologic sequelae of CMD and ultimately a clinical presentation with either shortness of breath, angina or both. Established causes for CMD in this setting are either an impaired coronary flow reserve/elevated microvascular resistance or coronary microvascular spasm [36]. Recently, detailed recommendations for the diagnosis of CMD in the clinic have been published [5], and a comprehensive assessment of both impaired vasodilatory capacity and assessment of enhanced vasoconstrictor responses to ACh has been recommended (so-called interventional diagnostic procedure, IDP) (Fig. 5.1).

Non-invasive assessments have revealed a prevalence of CMD between 26% and 54%. In the iPower study, 26% of 963 symptomatic women with no obstructive CAD had coronary flow velocity reserve <2 when assessed by transthoracic Doppler echo [23]. Furthermore, Murthy et al. [4] could show that PET-CFR was not only a powerful tool to diagnose CMD (prevalence ~50%), but that it can also be used as a powerful predictor of MACE since patients with a reduced CFR exhibited a higher likelihood of cardiovascular events.

Invasive assessment revealed that approximately 34% of patients with angina and unobstructed coronary arteries in the ACOVA study suffered from microvascular spasm (Fig. 5.3) [44] and approximately 50% of patients suffered from impaired CFR (Fig. 5.4) in another cohort as shown by Reis et al. [24]. The high prevalence of CMD in the setting of NOCAD has been recently confirmed in a study from the WISE cohort. The investigators compared their findings from coronary reactivity testing in an older patient cohort (1997–2001) with a more recent patient cohort (2009–2011) and endothelial and microvascular dysfunction prevalence and severity was similar to that found in the earlier original WISE cohort (overall approx. 40%) [46]. More recent data from Suda et al. have shown that when the IDP is applied in patients with angina and non-obstructive coronary arteries, 12% suffer from microvascular spasm, 35.3% suffer from impaired CFR, 40.1% suffer from a high IMR and 15% suffer from a combination of low CFR and high IMR [47]. These various forms of CMD are called endotypes and have been described in more

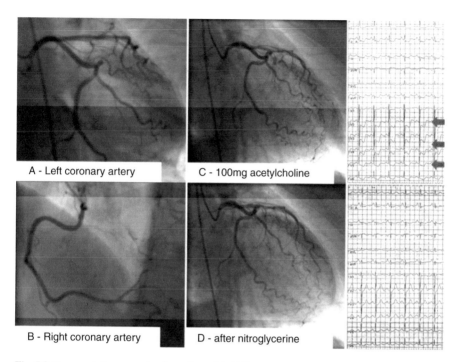

Fig. 5.3 Representative example of a patient with CMD, diagnosed with ACh provocation testing, as part of the IDP. This case presents a 73-year-old woman with hypercholesterolemia and recurrent attacks of resting angina pectoris associated with nausea and palpitations. Coronary angiography showed unobstructed but curly LCA (**a**). No relevant epicardial stenosis could be found in the RCA either (**b**). Additional intracoronary ACh testing to assess vasomotion in this patient revealed coronary microvascular spasm. The patient reported a reproduction of her usual symptoms and ST-segment depression in leads V2–V6 occurring at a dose of 100 mg of ACh (red arrows), without relevant epicardial vasoconstriction of the arteries (**c**). After intracoronary administration of nitroglycerine, her symptoms and ECG shifts quickly resolved (**d**). ACh, acetylcholine. (Reproduced from Ong et al. [5])

detail elsewhere [15]. A methodological limitation of the IDP is that CFR and microvascular resistance are often only measured in a single coronary artery (e.g. left anterior descending coronary artery) and not all three coronary arteries. This may be an important factor for the prevalence of CMD as studies could show that invasive evaluation of all three coronary arteries in 93 patients revealed 1-vessel CMD in 23.7% of cases, 2-vessel CMD in 14.0% and 3-vessel CMD in 3.2%. CMD was observed at a similar rate in the territories supplied by all three major coronary vessels (left anterior descending coronary artery 28.0%, left circumflex artery 19.4% and right coronary artery 23.7%; $P = 0.39$) [48].

Overall, the prevalence of CMD in patients with angina and unobstructed coronary arteries is not negligible and prospective randomized trials are on the way for the development of targeted treatments based on these different endotypes [16, 49]. Due to the high prevalence of CMD, additional assessments during invasive coronary angiography are highly recommended when epicardial disease is ruled out.

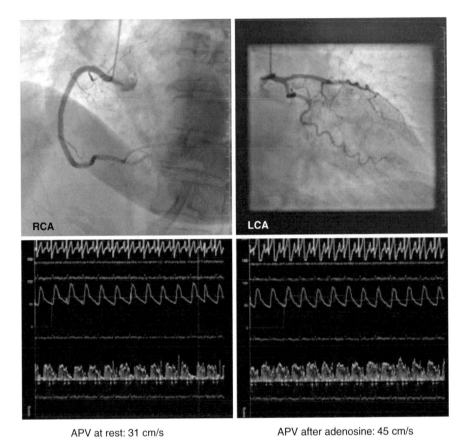

APV at rest: 31 cm/s   APV after adenosine: 45 cm/s

CFR = 1,5 → pathological

Fig. 5.4 Representative example of a patient with CMD, diagnosed with CFR measurement during IDP. This figure presents a case of a 74-year-old female patient with diabetes type 2, hypercholesterolemia, increased lipoprotein(a) and hypertension. She suffered from effort-related dyspnoea and chest tightness for several months. During coronary angiography, unobstructed coronary arteries could be seen (RCA and LCA). Additional CFR measurement in the left anterior descending coronary artery revealed a pathologically reduced CFR (1.5), indicating an impaired microvascular dilator capacity, which is known to be a typical long-term complication of diabetes affecting the coronary microvasculature. APV, average peak flow velocity. (Reproduced from Ong et al. [5])

5.8   Outlook

In times of personalized and individualized medicine, patients with angina and unobstructed coronary arteries should be comprehensively investigated (e.g. by an IDP). This is warranted because of the guarded prognosis of these patients in whom frequently the quality of life is severely impaired with loss of workforce in many cases. Indeed, studies by Jespersen et al. could show that the prevalence of persistent angina in patients with diffuse non-obstructive CAD or normal coronary arteries was higher compared to those with obstructive CAD [50, 51]. Moreover, patients with persistent angina were likely to suffer from long-term anxiety, depression, decrease in physical function and impairment of quality of life. Consequently, patients with angina symptoms and both obstructed or non-obstructed coronary arteries have a significantly higher likelihood of disability pension and premature workforce compared to the reference population [50, 51].

In patients with chest pain of unknown origin, novel smartphone-based ECG technologies offer a direct assessment of ischemic ECG changes during a chest pain attack [52]. This may reduce diagnostic uncertainty and prompt further diagnostic assessments. The broad applicability of this technology may also influence the epidemiology of CMD as many patients with chest pain of unknown origin may suffer from undetected CMD. Further studies are needed to provide robust data in this emerging field of digitalized medicine where artificial intelligence may also be involved.

Another important aspect is the female preponderance of patients with angina and unobstructed coronary arteries in general and those with CMD in particular [53]. Basic science as well as clinical research projects should focus on such sex differences and ensure equally distributed numbers of male and female study participants. It seems likely that individualized pharmacotherapy may also be different in male and female patients with CMD as recently shown in other cardiology drug studies [54]. Finally, research projects aiming at the discovery of systemic microvascular dysfunction and its associated conditions such as Raynaud's disease, cerebral microvascular dysfunction and microvascular renal impairment may revolutionize our understanding of CMD and put the condition in a new light [55].

5.9 Conclusion

CMD is an important condition often responsible for the clinical presentation of patients with angina and unobstructed coronary arteries. It can be comprehensively assessed by e.g. an interventional diagnostic procedure. The prevalence of CMD in patients with angina and unobstructed coronary arteries is high with approx. 50–60%. The unfavourable prognosis should prompt proper assessments enabling the treating physician to prescribe the most appropriate pharmacological treatment.

Acknowledgements The authors are grateful to Valeria Martínez Pereyra for her excellent support during the writing process of this chapter.

References

1. Camici PG, Crea F. Coronary microvascular dysfunction. N Engl J Med. 2007;356:830–40. https://doi.org/10.1056/NEJMra061889.

2. Chen C, Wei J, AlBadri A, Zarrini P, Bairey Merz CN. Coronary microvascular dysfunction – epidemiology, pathogenesis, prognosis, diagnosis, risk factors and therapy. Circ J. 2016;81:3–11. https://doi.org/10.1253/circj.CJ-16-1002.
3. Granger DN, Rodrigues SF, Yildirim A, Senchenkova EY. Microvascular responses to cardiovascular risk factors. Microcirculation. 2010;17:192–205. https://doi.org/10.1111/j.1549-8719.2009.00015.x.
4. Murthy VL, Naya M, Taqueti VR, Foster CR, Gaber M, Hainer J, Dorbala S, Blankstein R, Rimoldi O, Camici PG, Di Carli MF. Effects of sex on coronary microvascular dysfunction and cardiac outcomes. Circulation. 2014;129:2518–27. https://doi.org/10.1161/CIRCULATIONAHA.113.008507.
5. Ong P, Safdar B, Seitz A, Hubert A, Beltrame J, Prescott E. Diagnosis of coronary microvascular dysfunction in the clinic. Cardiovasc Res. 2020;116(4):841–55. https://doi.org/10.1093/cvr/cvz339.
6. Heberden W. Some account of a disorder of the breast. Med Trans R Col Phys. 1772;2:59–67.
7. Prinzmetal M, Kennamer R, Merliss R, Wada T, Bor N. Angina pectoris I. A variant form of angina pectoris. Am J Med. 1959;27:375–88. https://doi.org/10.1016/0002-9343(59)90003-8.
8. Proudfit WL, Bruschke AVG, Sones FM. Natural history of obstructive coronary artery disease: ten-year study of 601 nonsurgical cases. Prog Cardiovasc Dis. 1978;21:53–78. https://doi.org/10.1016/S0033-0620(78)80004-8.
9. Proudfit WL, Shirey EK, Sones FM. Selective cine coronary arteriography. Correlation with clinical findings in 1,000 patients. Circulation. 1966;33:901–10. https://doi.org/10.1161/01.cir.33.6.901.
10. Arbogast R, Bourassa MG. Myocardial function during atrial pacing in patients with angina pectoris and normal coronary arteriograms. Am J Cardiol. 1973;32:257–63. https://doi.org/10.1016/S0002-9149(73)80130-4.
11. Cannon RO, Epstein SE. "Microvascular angina" as a cause of chest pain with angiographically normal coronary arteries. Am J Cardiol. 1988;61:1338–43. https://doi.org/10.1016/0002-9149(88)91180-0.
12. Mohri M, Koyanagi M, Egashira K, Tagawa H, Ichiki T, Shimokawa H, Takeshita A. Angina pectoris caused by coronary microvascular spasm. Lancet. 1998;351:1165–9. https://doi.org/10.1016/S0140-6736(97)07329-7.
13. Sigwart U, Puel J, Mirkovitch V, Joffre F, Kappenberger L. Intravascular stents to prevent occlusion and restenosis after transluminal angioplasty. N Engl J Med. 1987;316:701–6. https://doi.org/10.1056/NEJM198703193161201.
14. Maseri A, editor. Ischemic heart disease: a rational basis for clinical practise and clinical research. New York: Churchill Livingstone; 1995.
15. Ford TJ, Berry C. How to diagnose and manage angina without obstructive coronary artery disease: lessons from the British Heart Foundation CorMicA trial. Interv Cardiol. 2019;14:76–82. https://doi.org/10.15420/icr.2019.04.R1.
16. Ford TJ, Stanley B, Good R, Rocchiccioli P, McEntegart M, Watkins S, Eteiba H, Shaukat A, Lindsay M, Robertson K, Hood S, McGeoch R, McDade R, Yii E, Sidik N, McCartney P, Corcoran D, Collison D, Rush C, McConnachie A, Touyz RM, Oldroyd KG, Berry C. Stratified medical therapy using invasive coronary function testing in angina: the CorMicA trial. J Am Coll Cardiol. 2018;72:2841–55. https://doi.org/10.1016/j.jacc.2018.09.006.
17. AlBadri A, Bairey Merz CN, Johnson BD, Wei J, Mehta PK, Cook-Wiens G, Reis SE, Kelsey SF, Bittner V, Sopko G, Shaw LJ, Pepine CJ, Ahmed B. Impact of abnormal coronary reactivity on long-term clinical outcomes in women. J Am Coll Cardiol. 2019;73:684–93. https://doi.org/10.1016/j.jacc.2018.11.040.
18. Wikipedia. Epidemiology - Wikipedia. 21.01.2020. https://en.wikipedia.org/w/index.php?oldid=936875258. Accessed 24 Jan 2020
19. Wikipedia. Inzidenz (Epidemiologie). 15.01.2020. https://de.wikipedia.org/w/index.php?oldid=194513835. Accessed 24 Jan 2020.

20. Wikipedia. Prävalenz. 15.01.2020. https://de.wikipedia.org/w/index.php?oldid=188357104. Accessed 24 Jan 2020.
21. Cassar A, Chareonthaitawee P, Rihal CS, Prasad A, Lennon RJ, Lerman LO, Lerman A. Lack of correlation between noninvasive stress tests and invasive coronary vasomotor dysfunction in patients with nonobstructive coronary artery disease. Circ Cardiovasc Interv. 2009;2:237–44. https://doi.org/10.1161/CIRCINTERVENTIONS.108.841056.
22. Hasdai D, Holmes DR, Higano ST, Burnett JC, Lerman A. Prevalence of coronary blood flow reserve abnormalities among patients with nonobstructive coronary artery disease and chest pain. Mayo Clin Proc. 1998;73:1133–40. https://doi.org/10.4065/73.12.1133.
23. Mygind ND, Michelsen MM, Pena A, Frestad D, Dose N, Aziz A, Faber R, Høst N, Gustafsson I, Hansen PR, Hansen HS, Bairey Merz CN, Kastrup J, Prescott E. Coronary microvascular function and cardiovascular risk factors in women with angina pectoris and no obstructive coronary artery disease: the iPOWER study. J Am Heart Assoc. 2016;5:e003064. https://doi.org/10.1161/JAHA.115.003064.
24. Reis SE, Holubkov R, Conrad Smith AJ, Kelsey SF, Sharaf BL, Reichek N, Rogers WJ, Merz CN, Sopko G, Pepine CJ. Coronary microvascular dysfunction is highly prevalent in women with chest pain in the absence of coronary artery disease: results from the NHLBI WISE study. Am Heart J. 2001;141:735–41. https://doi.org/10.1067/mhj.2001.114198.
25. Sade LE, Eroglu S, Bozbaş H, Ozbiçer S, Hayran M, Haberal A, Müderrisoğlu H. Relation between epicardial fat thickness and coronary flow reserve in women with chest pain and angiographically normal coronary arteries. Atherosclerosis. 2009;204:580–5. https://doi.org/10.1016/j.atherosclerosis.2008.09.038.
26. Sara JD, Widmer RJ, Matsuzawa Y, Lennon RJ, Lerman LO, Lerman A. Prevalence of coronary microvascular dysfunction among patients with chest pain and nonobstructive coronary artery disease. JACC Cardiovasc Interv. 2015;8:1445–53. https://doi.org/10.1016/j.jcin.2015.06.017.
27. Sicari R, Rigo F, Cortigiani L, Gherardi S, Galderisi M, Picano E. Additive prognostic value of coronary flow reserve in patients with chest pain syndrome and normal or near-normal coronary arteries. Am J Cardiol. 2009;103:626–31. https://doi.org/10.1016/j.amjcard.2008.10.033.
28. Wei J, Mehta PK, Johnson BD, Samuels B, Kar S, Anderson RD, Azarbal B, Petersen J, Sharaf B, Handberg E, Shufelt C, Kothawade K, Sopko G, Lerman A, Shaw L, Kelsey SF, Pepine CJ, Merz CNB. Safety of coronary reactivity testing in women with no obstructive coronary artery disease: results from the NHLBI-sponsored WISE (women's ischemia syndrome evaluation) study. JACC Cardiovasc Interv. 2012;5:646–53. https://doi.org/10.1016/j.jcin.2012.01.023.
29. Vermeltfoort IAC, Raijmakers PGHM, Riphagen II, Odekerken DAM, Kuijper AFM, Zwijnenburg A, Teule GJJ. Definitions and incidence of cardiac syndrome X: review and analysis of clinical data. Clin Res Cardiol. 2010;99:475–81. https://doi.org/10.1007/s00392-010-0159-1.
30. Bertrand ME, Lablanche JM, Bauters C, Leroy F, Mac FE. Discordant results of visual and quantitative estimates of stenosis severity before and after coronary angioplasty. Catheter Cardiovasc Diagn. 1993;28:1–6. https://doi.org/10.1002/ccd.1810280102.
31. Toth G, Hamilos M, Pyxaras S, Mangiacapra F, Nelis O, de Vroey F, Di Serafino L, Muller O, van Mieghem C, Wyffels E, Heyndrickx GR, Bartunek J, Vanderheyden M, Barbato E, Wijns W, de Bruyne B. Evolving concepts of angiogram: fractional flow reserve discordances in 4000 coronary stenoses. Eur Heart J. 2014;35:2831–8. https://doi.org/10.1093/eurheartj/ehu094.
32. Hoffmann U, Bamberg F, Chae CU, Nichols JH, Rogers IS, Seneviratne SK, Truong QA, Cury RC, Abbara S, Shapiro MD, Moloo J, Butler J, Ferencik M, Lee H, Jang I-K, Parry BA, Brown DF, Udelson JE, Achenbach S, Brady TJ, Nagurney JT. Coronary computed tomography angiography for early triage of patients with acute chest pain: the ROMICAT (rule out myocardial infarction using computer assisted tomography) trial. J Am Coll Cardiol. 2009;53:1642–50. https://doi.org/10.1016/j.jacc.2009.01.052.
33. Asher A, Singhal A, Thornton G, Wragg A, Davies C. FFRCT derived from computed tomography angiography: the experience in the UK. Expert Rev Cardiovasc Ther. 2018;16:919–29. https://doi.org/10.1080/14779072.2018.1538786.

34. Gonzalez JA, Lipinski MJ, Flors L, Shaw PW, Kramer CM, Salerno M. Meta-analysis of diagnostic performance of coronary computed tomography angiography, computed tomography perfusion, and computed tomography-fractional flow reserve in functional myocardial ischemia assessment versus invasive fractional flow reserve. Am J Cardiol. 2015;116:1469–78. https://doi.org/10.1016/j.amjcard.2015.07.078.

35. Sugisawa J, Matsumoto Y, Suda A, Ota H, Tsuchiya S, Ohyama K, Sato K, Shindo T, Ikeda S, Hao K, Kikuchi Y, Takahashi J, Shimokawa H. 1343Evidence for impaired vasodilator capacity of coronary microvessels in patients with vasospatic angina - myocardial CT perfusion imaging study. Eur Heart J. 2018;39(suppl_1). https://doi.org/10.1093/eurheartj/ehy565.1343.

36. Ong P, Camici PG, Beltrame JF, Crea F, Shimokawa H, Sechtem U, Kaski JC, Bairey Merz CN. International standardization of diagnostic criteria for microvascular angina. Int J Cardiol. 2018;250:16–20. https://doi.org/10.1016/j.ijcard.2017.08.068.

37. Hochman JS, Tamis JE, Thompson TD, Weaver WD, White HD, van de Werf F, Aylward P, Topol EJ, Califf RM. Sex, clinical presentation, and outcome in patients with acute coronary syndromes. Global use of strategies to open occluded coronary arteries in acute coronary syndromes IIb investigators. N Engl J Med. 1999;341:226–32. https://doi.org/10.1056/NEJM199907223410402.

38. Pasupathy S, Air T, Dreyer RP, Tavella R, Beltrame JF. Systematic review of patients presenting with suspected myocardial infarction and nonobstructive coronary arteries. Circulation. 2015;131:861–70. https://doi.org/10.1161/CIRCULATIONAHA.114.011201.

39. Tamis-Holland JE, Jneid H, Reynolds HR, Agewall S, Brilakis ES, Brown TM, Lerman A, Cushman M, Kumbhani DJ, Arslanian-Engoren C, Bolger AF, Beltrame JF. Contemporary diagnosis and management of patients with myocardial infarction in the absence of obstructive coronary artery disease: a scientific statement from the American Heart Association. Circulation. 2019;139:e891–908. https://doi.org/10.1161/CIR.0000000000000670.

40. Safdar B, D'Onofrio G, Dziura J, Russell RR, Johnson C, Sinusas AJ. Prevalence and characteristics of coronary microvascular dysfunction among chest pain patients in the emergency department. Eur Heart J Acute Cardiovasc Care. 2020;9(1):5–13. https://doi.org/10.1177/2048872618764418.

41. Sato K, Kaikita K, Nakayama N, Horio E, Yoshimura H, Ono T, Ohba K, Tsujita K, Kojima S, Tayama S, Hokimoto S, Matsui K, Sugiyama S, Yamabe H, Ogawa H. Coronary vasomotor response to intracoronary acetylcholine injection, clinical features, and long-term prognosis in 873 consecutive patients with coronary spasm: analysis of a single-center study over 20 years. J Am Heart Assoc. 2013;2:e000227. https://doi.org/10.1161/JAHA.113.000227.

42. Pirozzolo G, Seitz A, Athanasiadis A, Bekeredjian R, Sechtem U, Ong P. Microvascular spasm in non-ST-segment elevation myocardial infarction without culprit lesion (MINOCA). Clin Res Cardiol. 2020;109(2):246–54. https://doi.org/10.1007/s00392-019-01507-w.

43. Patel MR, Peterson ED, Dai D, Brennan JM, Redberg RF, Anderson HV, Brindis RG, Douglas PS. Low diagnostic yield of elective coronary angiography. N Engl J Med. 2010;362:886–95. https://doi.org/10.1056/NEJMoa0907272.

44. Ong P, Athanasiadis A, Borgulya G, Mahrholdt H, Kaski JC, Sechtem U. High prevalence of a pathological response to acetylcholine testing in patients with stable angina pectoris and unobstructed coronary arteries. The ACOVA study (Abnormal COronary VAsomotion in patients with stable angina and unobstructed coronary arteries). J Am Coll Cardiol. 2012;59:655–62. https://doi.org/10.1016/j.jacc.2011.11.015.

45. Jespersen L, Hvelplund A, Abildstrøm SZ, Pedersen F, Galatius S, Madsen JK, Jørgensen E, Kelbæk H, Prescott E. Stable angina pectoris with no obstructive coronary artery disease is associated with increased risks of major adverse cardiovascular events. Eur Heart J. 2012;33:734–44. https://doi.org/10.1093/eurheartj/ehr331.

46. Anderson RD, Petersen JW, Mehta PK, Wei J, Johnson BD, Handberg EM, Kar S, Samuels B, Azarbal B, Kothawade K, Kelsey SF, Sharaf B, Shaw LJ, Sopko G, Bairey Merz CN, Pepine CJ. Prevalence of coronary endothelial and microvascular dysfunction in women with symptoms of ischemia and no obstructive coronary artery disease is confirmed by a new cohort: The

NHLBI-sponsored women's ischemia syndrome evaluation-coronary vascular dysfunction (WISE-CVD). J Interv Cardiol. 2019;2019:7169275. https://doi.org/10.1155/2019/7169275.

47. Suda A, Takahashi J, Hao K, Kikuchi Y, Shindo T, Ikeda S, Sato K, Sugisawa J, Matsumoto Y, Miyata S, Sakata Y, Shimokawa H. Coronary functional abnormalities in patients with angina and nonobstructive coronary artery disease. J Am Coll Cardiol. 2019;74:2350–60. https://doi.org/10.1016/j.jacc.2019.08.1056.

48. Kobayashi Y, Lee JM, Fearon WF, Lee JH, Nishi T, Choi D-H, Zimmermann FM, Jung J-H, Lee H-J, Doh J-H, Nam C-W, Shin E-S, Koo B-K. Three-vessel assessment of coronary microvascular dysfunction in patients with clinical suspicion of ischemia: prospective observational study with the index of microcirculatory resistance. Circ Cardiovasc Interv. 2018;11(2):e006262. https://doi.org/10.1161/CIRCINTERVENTIONS.117.005445.

49. Ford TJ, Stanley B, Sidik N, Good R, Rocchiccioli P, McEntegart M, Watkins S, Eteiba H, Shaukat A, Lindsay M, Robertson K, Hood S, McGeoch R, McDade R, Yii E, McCartney P, Corcoran D, Collison D, Rush C, Sattar N, McConnachie A, Touyz RM, Oldroyd KG, Berry C. 1-year outcomes of angina management guided by invasive coronary function testing (CorMicA). JACC Cardiovasc Interv. 2020;13:33–45. https://doi.org/10.1016/j.jcin.2019.11.001.

50. Jespersen L, Abildstrøm SZ, Hvelplund A, Prescott E. Persistent angina: highly prevalent and associated with long-term anxiety, depression, low physical functioning, and quality of life in stable angina pectoris. Clin Res Cardiol. 2013;102:571–81. https://doi.org/10.1007/s00392-013-0568-z.

51. Jespersen L, Abildstrøm SZ, Hvelplund A, Galatius S, Madsen JK, Pedersen F, Højberg S, Prescott E. Symptoms of angina pectoris increase the probability of disability pension and premature exit from the workforce even in the absence of obstructive coronary artery disease. Eur Heart J. 2013;34:3294–303. https://doi.org/10.1093/eurheartj/eht395.

52. Bonaventura K, Wellnhofer E, Fleck E. Comparison of standard and derived 12-lead electro-cardiograms registrated by a simplified 3-lead setting with four electrodes for diagnosis of coronary angioplasty-induced myocardial ischemia. Eur Cardiol. 2012;8(3):179.

53. Aziz A, Hansen HS, Sechtem U, Prescott E, Ong P. Sex-related differences in vasomotor function in patients with angina and unobstructed coronary arteries. J Am Coll Cardiol. 2017;70:2349–58. https://doi.org/10.1016/j.jacc.2017.09.016.

54. Solomon SD, JJV MM, Anand IS, Ge J, CSP L, Maggioni AP, Martinez F, Packer M, Pfeffer MA, Pieske B, Redfield MM, Rouleau JL, van Veldhuisen DJ, Zannad F, Zile MR, Desai AS, Claggett B, Jhund PS, Boytsov SA, Comin-Colet J, Cleland J, Düngen H-D, Goncalvesova E, Katova T, Kerr Saraiva JF, Lelonek M, Merkely B, Senni M, Shah SJ, Zhou J, Rizkala AR, Gong J, Shi VC, Lefkowitz MP. Angiotensin-neprilysin inhibition in heart failure with preserved ejection fraction. N Engl J Med. 2019;381:1609–20. https://doi.org/10.1056/NEJMoa1908655.

55. Ford TJ, Rocchiccioli P, Good R, McEntegart M, Eteiba H, Watkins S, Shaukat A, Lindsay M, Robertson K, Hood S, Yii E, Sidik N, Harvey A, Montezano AC, Beattie E, Haddow L, Oldroyd KG, Touyz RM, Berry C. Systemic microvascular dysfunction in microvascular and vasospastic angina. Eur Heart J. 2018;39:4086–97. https://doi.org/10.1093/eurheartj/ehy529.

Chapter 6
Pathophysiology of Coronary Microvascular Dysfunction

Shigeo Godo and Hiroaki Shimokawa

Abstract Coronary microvascular dysfunction (CMD) has been implicated in a wide spectrum of cardiovascular disease. The underlying mechanisms of CMD appear to be heterogeneous, including several structural and functional alterations. Among them, central to coronary vasomotion abnormalities are threefold: enhanced coronary vasoconstrictive reactivity (i.e. coronary spasm) at epicardial and microvascular levels, reduced endothelium-dependent and -independent coronary vasodilator capacity, and increased coronary microvascular resistance, all of which can cause myocardial ischemia due to CMD and often coexist in various combinations even in the absence of obstructive coronary artery disease. The endothelium plays essential roles in modulating vascular tone by synthesizing and releasing endothelium-derived relaxing factors, including vasodilator prostaglandins, nitric oxide (NO), and endothelium-dependent hyperpolarization (EDH) factors in a distinct vessel size–dependent manner; NO mainly mediates vasodilatation of relatively large, conduit vessels (e.g. epicardial coronary arteries), while EDH factors in small resistance vessels (e.g. coronary microvessels). Endothelium-derived hydrogen peroxide (H_2O_2) is a physiological signaling molecule serving as one of the major EDH factors especially in coronary microcirculation and has gained increasing attention in view of its emerging relevance for cardiovascular disease. In this chapter, we will briefly summarize the latest knowledge on the pathophysiology of CMD with a special reference to endothelial modulation of vascular tone mediated by H_2O_2/EDH factor and coronary microvascular spasm, in addition to discussing clinical implications of and therapeutic approaches to CMD in cardiovascular disease.

Keywords Coronary microvascular dysfunction · Endothelial function · Endothelium-dependent hyperpolarization · Nitric oxide · Hydrogen peroxide

S. Godo · H. Shimokawa (✉)
Department of Cardiovascular Medicine, Tohoku University Graduate School of Medicine, Sendai, Miyagi, Japan
e-mail: shimo@cardio.med.tohoku.ac.jp

© Springer Nature Singapore Pte Ltd. 2021
H. Shimokawa (ed.), *Coronary Vasomotion Abnormalities*,
https://doi.org/10.1007/978-981-15-7594-5_6

Abbreviations

CAD	Coronary artery disease
cGMP	Cyclic guanosine monophosphate
CMD	Coronary microvascular dysfunction
EDH	Endothelium-dependent hyperpolarization
EDRF(s)	Endothelium-derived relaxing factor(s)
EETs	Epoxyeicosatrienoic acids
eNOS	Endothelial nitric oxide synthase
H_2O_2	Hydrogen peroxide
HFpEF	Heart failure with preserved ejection fraction
IHD	Ischemic heart disease
INOCA	Ischemia and no obstructive coronary artery disease
NO	Nitric oxide
NOS	Nitric oxide synthase
PGs	Prostaglandins
PKG	cGMP-dependent protein kinase
ROS	Reactive oxygen species
sGC	Soluble guanylate cyclase
SOD	Superoxide dismutase
VSMC	Vascular smooth muscle cells

6.1   Introduction

A growing body of evidence has demonstrated that coronary microvascular dysfunction (CMD) plays important roles in the pathophysiology of cardiac ischemia in patients with a wide spectrum of cardiovascular disorders, including ischemic heart disease (IHD) [1, 2], aortic stenosis [3], and heart failure with preserved ejection fraction (HFpEF) [4–6]. More than 50% of patients undergoing invasive coronary angiography for the evaluation of suspected obstructive coronary artery disease (CAD) have no significant coronary artery stenosis [7], where the role of CMD has been recognized as an alternative mechanism for symptoms and signs of myocardial ischemia. Indeed, recent studies using comprehensive assessment of coronary physiology by multimodality protocols have unveiled that a substantial proportion of patients with ischemia and no obstructive coronary artery disease (INOCA) differ in the underlying coronary microvascular physiology [8–11]. Mechanistically, structural and functional abnormalities of "epicardial" coronary arteries in patients with IHD are the focus of previous studies; however, those of coronary microvasculature, referred to as CMD, have attracted much attention in view of their unexpectedly high prevalence in and significant prognostic impact on this population in many clinical settings [12–14]. The etiologies of CMD appear to be heterogeneous; several structural (e.g. luminal obstruction, vascular remodeling, vascular rarefaction, and extramural compression) and functional alterations (e.g. endothelial dysfunction, vascular smooth muscle cells [VSMC] dysfunction, and microvascular spasm) have been proposed for the pathophysiological mechanisms of CMD [15–19]. Among them, central to coronary vasomotion abnormalities [1, 20] are enhanced coronary vasoconstrictive reactivity (i.e. coronary spasm) not only at epicardial but also at microvascular levels, reduced endothelium-dependent and -independent coronary vasodilator capacity (e.g. coronary flow reserve [CFR] <2.0), and increased coronary microvascular resistance (e.g. index of microvascular resistance [IMR] >25), all of which can cause myocardial ischemia due to CMD even in the absence of obstructive CAD and often coexist in various combinations in patients with angina and non-obstructive CAD [8, 10, 11].

In this chapter, we will briefly summarize the current knowledge on the pathophysiology of CMD with a special reference to endothelial modulation of vascular tone and coronary microvascular spasm, in addition to briefly discussing clinical implications of and therapeutic approaches to CMD in cardiovascular disease. Further discussions on the coronary microcirculation physiology are available elsewhere [15–19, 21, 22].

6.2 Endothelial Modulation of Vascular Tone: NO and EDH Factors

6.2.1 Vessel Size–Dependent Contribution of Endothelium-Derived Relaxing Factors

The endothelium plays pivotal roles in modulating the tone of underlying VSMC by synthesizing and releasing endothelium-derived relaxing factors (EDRFs) in an autocrine and paracrine manner, including vasodilator prostaglandins (PGs) (e.g. prostacyclin), nitric oxide (NO), and endothelium-dependent hyperpolarization (EDH) factors, as well as endothelium-derived contracting factors [1, 23, 24] (Fig. 6.1). Endothelial dysfunction is characterized by reduced production and/or action of EDRFs, serving as the hallmark of atherosclerotic cardiovascular diseases as well as one of the major pathogenetic mechanisms of CMD [15–18]. Of note is that these EDRFs regulate vascular tone in a distinct vessel size–dependent fashion [25, 26] (Fig. 6.1); endothelium-derived NO mainly mediates vasodilatation of relatively large, conduit vessels (e.g. epicardial coronary arteries), while EDH factors-mediated responses are the predominant mechanisms of endothelium-dependent vasodilatation of resistance arteries (e.g. coronary microvessels). By contrast, vasodilator PGs play a small but constant role in general, independent of vessel size. This vessel-size-dependent contribution of NO and EDH factors in endothelium-dependent vasodilatation is well preserved from

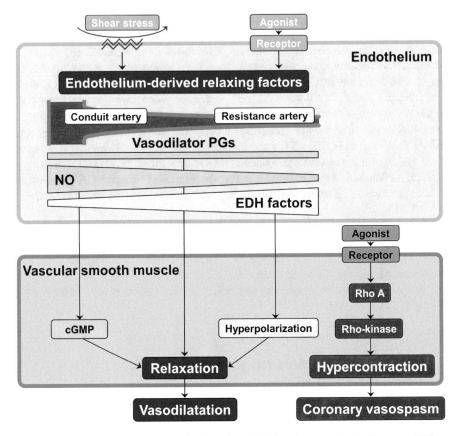

Fig. 6.1 Vessel size–dependent contribution of endothelium-derived relaxing factors and Rho-kinase-mediated vascular smooth muscle hypercontraction. *cGMP* cyclic guanosine monophosphate, *EDH* endothelium-dependent hyperpolarization, *NO* nitric oxide, *PGs* prostaglandins. (Reproduced from Shimokawa and Godo [24])

rodents to humans, shaping a physiological balance between them [1, 23]. Thus, EDH factors-mediated vasodilatation is a vital mechanism especially in microcirculations, where blood pressure and organ perfusion are critically determined. Moreover, such redundant mechanisms in endothelium-dependent vasodilatations are advantageous for ensuring proper maintenance of vascular tone under pathological conditions, where one of EDRFs-mediated responses is impaired, favoring a vasoconstrictor and proinflammatory state. Indeed, in various pathological conditions with atherosclerotic risk factors, NO-mediated relaxations are easily compromised, while EDH factors-mediated responses are fairly preserved or even enhanced to serve as a compensatory vasodilator system [26, 27]. Multiple mechanisms are involved in the enhanced EDH factors-mediated responses in small resistance vessels, including negative interactions between NO and several EDH factors, as discussed later. The regulatory mechanisms of NO-mediated responses are extensively reviewed elsewhere [28–30].

6.2.2 EDH Factors: The Predominant Mechanism of Vasodilatation in Small Arteries

In 1998, Feletou and Vanhoutte [31] and Chen et al. [32] independently demonstrated the existence of endothelium-derived non-NO, non-prostanoid relaxing factors, unforeseen EDH factors. EDH factors-mediated responses are the major mechanism of endothelium-dependent vasodilatations in resistance arteries, although, by definition, the contribution of EDH factors is determined only after the blockade of both vasodilator PGs and NO. EDH factors cause hyperpolarization and subsequent relaxation of underlying VSMC with resultant vasodilatation of small resistance vessels and thus finely regulate blood pressure and organ perfusion instantaneously in response to diverse physiological demands [23, 33]. The nature of EDH factors varies depending on the vascular bed, vessel size, and species of interest, including epoxyeicosatrienoic acids (EETs), metabolites of arachidonic P450 epoxygenase pathway [34, 35], electrical communication through gap junctions [36], K^+ ions [37], and as we demonstrated, endothelium-derived hydrogen peroxide (H_2O_2) [24, 38] (Fig. 6.2). EETs

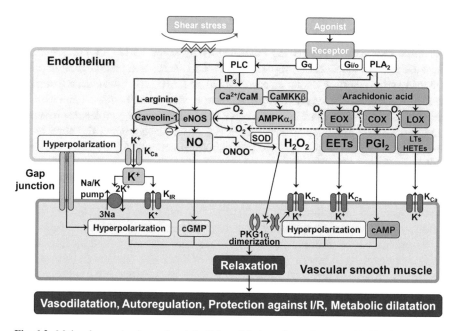

Fig. 6.2 Molecular mechanisms of endothelial modulation of vascular tone. *AMPKα1* α1-subunit of AMP-activated protein kinase, *CaM* calmodulin, *CaMKKβ* Ca^{2+}/CaM-dependent protein kinase β, *cAMP* cyclic AMP, *cGMP* cyclic GMP, *COX* cyclooxygenase, *EETs* epoxyeicosatrienoic acids, *eNOS* endothelial NO synthase, *EOX* epoxygenase, *HETEs* hydroxyeicosatetraenoic acids, *H₂O₂* hydrogen peroxide, *IP₃* inositol trisphosphate, *I/R* ischemia-reperfusion injury, K_{Ca} calcium-activated potassium channel, K_{IR} inwardly rectifying potassium channel, *LOX* lipoxygenase, *LTs* leukotrienes, *NO* nitric oxide, *ONOO⁻* peroxynitrite, *PGI₂* prostacyclin, *PKG1α* 1α-subunit of protein kinase G, *PLA₂* phospholipase A_2, *PLC* phospholipase C, *SOD* superoxide dismutase. (Reproduced from Shimokawa and Godo [24])

mainly participate in EDH-mediated relaxations in bovine [34], porcine [35], and human coronary arteries [39]; K$^+$ ions in rat hepatic and mesenteric arteries [37, 40], porcine [41] and bovine [42] coronary arteries, and human kidney interlobar arteries [43]; and H$_2$O$_2$, at physiologically low concentrations, in human [44], porcine [45], and canine coronary arteries [46–48].

Coronary vascular resistance is predominantly determined by the pre-arterioles (>100 μm in diameter) and arterioles (<100 μm) where EDH factors-mediated responses become more prominent than NO-mediated relaxations. Given that H$_2$O$_2$ has potent vasodilator properties in coronary resistance vessels, impaired H$_2$O$_2$-mediated vasodilatation may lead to CMD. In the next section, we will focus on endothelium-derived H$_2$O$_2$ as an EDH factor in detail. Readers are encouraged to refer to an excellent textbook for more comprehensive information on the role of other EDH factors [49].

6.3 Endothelium-Derived H$_2$O$_2$ as an EDH Factor

6.3.1 Identification of H$_2$O$_2$/EDH Factor

Reactive oxygen species (ROS) have been considered to be primarily harmful because of their detrimental property to cells and tissues and pathological implications in various cardiovascular diseases including CMD [50]. However, as exemplified by endothelium-derived H$_2$O$_2$/EDH factor, many studies have demonstrated that physiological levels of ROS can serve as crucial signaling molecules in health and disease [51] and have acknowledged H$_2$O$_2$ as a physiological signaling molecule, regulating blood pressure [52], metabolic functions [53, 54], and coronary microcirculation [46–48].

Following the original reports on the existence of EDH factors in 1988 [31, 32], we hypothesized that a putative EDH factor might be a non-NO vasodilator substance (likely ROS) derived from endothelial NO synthases (NOSs) system, based on a hint from several early observations and notions. First, both NO-mediated and EDH-mediated responses are susceptible to vascular injuries caused by atherosclerotic risk factors, and inversely, the treatment of those risk factors can restore both responses [1, 26]. Second, it had been previously demonstrated that endothelium-derived free radicals exert endothelium-dependent vasodilator and vasoconstrictor effects in canine coronary arteries [55]. Third, both endothelial NOS (eNOS)-derived NO generation and EDH-mediated responses are dependent on calcium/calmodulin [56]. Fourth, a simple molecule (like NO), rather than complex substances, may be opportune for modulating vascular tone instantaneously in response to various physiological demands in the body. On the basis of these notions, in 2000, we demonstrated for the first time that endothelium-derived H$_2$O$_2$ is an EDH factor in mouse mesenteric arteries; EDH-mediated hyperpolarizations and relaxations of underlying VSMC were inhibited by catalase, a specific H$_2$O$_2$ inhibitor, in small mesenteric arteries from wild-type mice and were significantly reduced in eNOS-knockout (KO) mice [38]. This was also true for other vascular beds, including human mesenteric [57] and coronary [58] arteries, porcine [45] and canine [46–48] coronary arteries, and piglet pial arterioles [59]. Notably, the estimated concentrations of endothelium-derived H_2O_2/EDH factor are in micromolar order (<50 μmol/L) [45, 47], which are much lower concentrations than those observed in various pathological conditions [60]. When applied in organ chamber experiments, approximately 10–100 μmol/L of exogenous H_2O_2 elicits vasodilatation of human coronary arterioles [58, 61] and mouse small mesenteric arteries [38, 62, 63], while higher concentrations of H_2O_2 rather induce vasoconstriction by releasing cyclooxygenase-derived thromboxane [64]. Here, only 10–15% of H_2O_2 applied exogenously reaches the intracellular targets due to endogenous antioxidants and membrane impedance [65].

6.3.2 Source of H_2O_2/EDH Factor

Endothelium-derived H_2O_2 is mainly produced by the dismutation of superoxide anions derived from various sources in the endothelium, including NADPH oxidase, mitochondrial electron transport chain, xanthine oxidase, lipoxygenase, and NOSs (Fig. 6.2) [60]. Importantly, superoxide anions relevant to H_2O_2/EDH factor are not derived from pathologically uncoupled eNOS because H_2O_2-mediated EDH-type responses are not cancelled by NOS inhibitors (i.e. L-arginine analogs) and upregulation of eNOS co-factor tetrahydrobiopterin has no effects on the responses [66]. eNOS produces superoxide anions under physiological conditions when synthesizing NO from L-arginine and oxygen, while Cu,Zn-SOD dismutates those superoxide anions into H_2O_2. Cu,Zn-SOD-KO mice show markedly impaired EDH-mediated hyperpolarizations and relaxations in mesenteric arteries and coronary circulation without VSMC dysfunction [67]. Other sources of superoxide anions in H_2O_2-mediated vasodilatation have been identified in human coronary arterioles, including mitochondrial respiratory chain in flow-mediated dilatation [68] and NADPH oxidase in bradykinin-induced relaxation [69].

6.3.3 Regulatory Mechanisms of Physiologically Relevant H_2O_2

Recent studies have provided potential regulatory mechanisms underlying the physiologically relevant H_2O_2 in the endothelium [51]. It is important to note that local subcellular concentrations at microdomains, rather than net cellular concentrations, may be critical to determine whether the effects of ROS can be detrimental or beneficial for cellular signaling and that co-localization of the source and target of H_2O_2

may help to avoid non-specific harmful oxidations [70, 71]. In addition, specific cysteine residues, such as peroxiredoxins, can function as a redox-dependent molecular switch to regulate ROS-mediated signaling [60]. Moreover, a novel mechanism of CMD in human CAD has been proposed [22, 72, 73]. As mentioned above, healthy human coronary circulation is regulated by NO and low physiological levels of H_2O_2/EDH factor. However, various atherosclerotic risk factors (e.g. aging, hypertension, obesity, and smoking) can cause a switch from NO to H_2O_2 in the mediator of endothelium-dependent vasodilatation in human coronary arteries. The resultant impaired production of NO and pathologically elevated levels of H_2O_2 manifest as CMD that favors a vasoconstrictor and pro-inflammatory state, leading to the development of coronary atherosclerosis [22, 72, 73].

6.3.4   Mode of Action of H_2O_2/EDH Factor

Among several modes of action of H_2O_2/EDH factor [74, 75], oxidative modification of cGMP-dependent protein kinase (PKG) plays a central role in H_2O_2-induced hyperpolarization and relaxation of underlying VSMC [52, 76] (Fig. 6.2). Briefly, H_2O_2 induces dimerization of 1α-isoforms of PKG (PKG1α) through an interprotein disulfide bond formation between them to enhance the kinase activity through phosphorylation. The activated PKG1α subsequently stimulates K^+ channels with resultant hyperpolarization and vasodilatation in mouse mesenteric arteries [52] and human coronary arterioles [58, 61]. H_2O_2 also promotes the translocation of PKG1α from cytoplasm to membrane in human [61] and porcine [77] coronary arteries. Such reversible post-translational modification, like phosphorylation, is advantageous for the fine control of vascular tone in response to various demand fluctuation in vivo [30].

6.3.5   Clinical Significance of H_2O_2/EDH Factor

The oxidant-mediated signaling by H_2O_2 is of clinical importance because it is associated with blood pressure control in vivo [52]. Pharmacological inhibition of catalase decreases arterial blood pressure in association with enhanced PKG1α dimerization in vivo [77]. Moreover, the 'redox-dead' knock-in mice of Cys42Ser PKG1α, whose mutant PKG1α is unable to be activated by H_2O_2-induced dimerization because of the deletion in its redox-sensitive sulfur, exhibit markedly impaired EDH-mediated hyperpolarization and relaxation in resistance arteries ex vivo associated with systemic arterial hypertension [52]. Furthermore, physiological levels of H_2O_2 have potent vasodilator properties in coronary resistance vessels, contributing to coronary autoregulation [46], cardioprotection against myocardial ischemia-reperfusion injury [47], and tachycardia-induced metabolic coronary vasodilatations [48] in dogs in vivo. Given that coronary vascular resistance is predominantly determined by the prearterioles and arterioles [17] where the effect of EDH-mediated responses on vascular tone is superior to that of NO-mediated relaxations, it is important to maintain the vessel size–dependent contribution of NO and EDH factors for the treatment of CMD. Taken together, endothelium-derived H_2O_2 functions as an important endogenous second messenger at its physiological low concentrations to elicit EDH-mediated vasodilatation and to maintain vascular homeostasis in the coronary circulation [23, 74]. In the clinical settings, it has been repeatedly reported that the effects of chronic nitrate therapy are neutral or even harmful in patients with cardiovascular diseases [78–82] and that antioxidant treatments are disappointingly ineffective to prevent cardiovascular events [83]. These lines of evidence suggest the importance of the physiological balance between NO and H_2O_2/EDH factor in maintaining cardiovascular homeostasis and in curing diseases associated with endothelial dysfunction.

6.4 Mechanisms of Enhanced H_2O_2/EDH Factor in Microcirculation

6.4.1 Diverse Roles of Endothelial NOSs System

Endothelium-derived NO and EDH factors share the roles in modulating vascular tone in a distinct vessel size–dependent manner through the diverse roles of endothelial NOSs system (Fig. 6.2). In large conduit vessels, NOSs mainly act as a NO-generating system to cause soluble guanylate cyclase (sGC)-cyclic guanosine monophosphate (cGMP)-mediated vasodilatation, whereas in small resistance vessels, they serve as a superoxide-generating system to evoke H_2O_2/EDH factor-mediated responses [84]. Among three NOS isoforms (neural NOS [nNOS, NOS1], inducible NOS [iNOS, NOS2], and eNOS, NOS3) expressed in the cardiovascular system, eNOS is the dominant isoform in blood vessels [85] and the most important isoform in generating H_2O_2/EDH factor in the endothelium [86]. As mentioned above, genetic ablation of eNOS in mice results in impaired EDH-mediated vasodilatation associated with systemic hypertension [87]. Using singly-eNOS-KO, doubly-n/eNOS-KO, and triply-n/i/eNOS-KO mice, we have previously demonstrated that EDH-mediated relaxations are progressively reduced in accordance with the number of NOS genes ablated [84]. As compared with wild-type mice, H_2O_2-mediated EDH-type relaxations of small mesenteric arteries are reduced approximately by half in singly-eNOS-KO mice, further diminished in doubly-n/eNOS-KO mice, and are finally absent in triply-n/i/eNOS-KO mice without underlying VSMC dysfunction [84]. The remaining EDH-mediated relaxation of small mesenteric arteries in eNOS-KO mice is still sensitive to catalase [38]. Collectively, these results indicate that three NOSs isoforms compensate each other to maintain H_2O_2-mediated EDH-type relaxations.

6.4.2 Mechanisms for H_2O_2/EDH Factor Dominance in Coronary Microcirculation

Accumulating evidence has provided mechanistic insights into vessel size–dependent contribution of NO and H_2O_2/EDH factor in coronary microcirculation. Pretreatment with NO donors attenuates EDH-mediated vasodilatation in porcine coronary arteries in vitro [88] and canine coronary microcirculation in vivo [89] and NO exerts a negative-feedback effect on endothelium-dependent vasodilatation through cGMP-mediated desensitization in canine coronary arteries ex vivo [90]. Mechanistically, cGMP-dependent activation of PKG desensitizes VSMC to H_2O_2 by inhibiting H_2O_2-induced PKG1α dimerization, a central mechanism of H_2O_2/EDH factor-mediated vasodilatation, and conversely, pharmacological inhibition of sGC sensitizes conduit vessels, but not resistance vessels, to H_2O_2-induced vasodilatation in mice [91]. In addition, mouse resistance vessels have less NO production and less antioxidant capacity, predisposing PKG1α to be more sensitive to H_2O_2-induced activation [91]. Other key players for enhanced H_2O_2/EDH factor-mediated vasodilatation in coronary microcirculation include endothelial caveolin-1, a negative regulator of eNOS [62, 92], and α1-subunit of endothelial AMP-activated protein kinase [93]. Taken together, these mechanisms are compatible with the widely held view that EDH-mediated responses function as a compensatory vasodilator system when NO-mediated relaxations are compromised. It is important to maintain the vessel size–dependent contribution of NO and EDH factors because excessive endothelial NO production by either caveolin-1 deficiency or eNOS overexpression disrupts the physiological balance between NO and EDH factors in endothelium-dependent vasodilatation, compromising coronary flow reserve in mice in vivo [63, 92].

6.5 Coronary Microvascular Spasm

Besides endothelial dysfunction, CMD can be caused by endothelium-independent mechanisms in general, which encompass impaired coronary microvascular dilatation and enhanced coronary microvascular constriction. Coronary artery spasms at both epicardial and microvascular levels have been implicated in a wide variety of IHD [1]. Mechanistically, Rho-kinase-induced myosin light chain phosphorylation with resultant VSMC hypercontraction is the central mechanism in the pathogenesis of coronary artery spasm at epicardial [94, 95] as well as at microvascular [96] levels, whereas the role of endothelial dysfunction may be minimal (Fig. 6.1) [1, 20]. Intracoronary administration of a Rho-kinase inhibitor, fasudil, is effective not only for relieving refractory coronary spasm resistant to nitrates or calcium-channel blockers but also for suppressing coronary microvascular spasm in most patients with the disorder [97]. In addition, enhanced epicardial and coronary microvascular spasms are associated with increased production of other vasoconstrictive mediators, such as endothelin [98] and serotonin [99] in patients with CMD.

Intracoronary acetylcholine (ACh) provocation test is useful in inducing coronary artery spasm with high sensitivity and specificity in the cardiac catheter laboratory [100]. A high prevalence of ACh-induced coronary microvascular spasm has been reported in one-third of patients with stable chest pain and non-obstructive CAD [101, 102]. The Coronary Vasomotion Disorders International Study (COVADIS) Group proposed a consensus set of standardized diagnostic criteria for microvascular angina attributable to CMD, including ACh-induced coronary microvascular spasm [103]. The diagnostic value of these criteria has been demonstrated by a recent randomized clinical trial [104]. More recently, we have demonstrated that increased coronary microvascular resistance as evaluated by IMR is associated with Rho-kinase activation in the pathogenesis of coronary functional abnormalities [11]. Considering that patients with coronary artery spasm are not necessarily associated with conventional coronary risk factors and positive results of non-invasive functional stress tests, comprehensive assessment of coronary physiology using multimodality protocol is of diagnostic value to identify coronary vasomotion abnormalities and to avoid false reassurance in patients with INOCA [10, 11, 100].

6.6 Clinical Implications

6.6.1 Importance of Endothelial Function Tests

Assessment of endothelial function has been acknowledged as an excellent surrogate marker of future cardiovascular events in many clinical settings [105], although it is challenging to specifically assess EDH factors-mediated responses in humans in vivo. The reason for this difficulty is at least twofold: (1) the contribution of EDH factors could be determined only after the blockade of both vasodilator PGs and NO and (2) coronary resistance arteries are not visible on coronary angiography. Endothelial dysfunction is manifested as impaired production and/or action of EDRFs. EDH factors-mediated vasodilation can be temporarily enhanced to compensate for impaired NO-mediated responses in the early stage of atherosclerotic conditions [33, 74]. However, after prolonged exposure to atherosclerotic risk factors, this compensatory role of EDH factors-mediated responses is finally disrupted to cause metabolic disturbance [106]. Endothelial dysfunction, as evaluated by impaired flow-mediated dilation (FMD) of the brachial artery or digital reactive hyperemia index (RHI) in peripheral arterial tonometry, is associated with future cardiovascular events in patients with CAD and one standard deviation decrease in FMD or RHI is associated with doubling of cardiovascular event risk [105]. More recently, peripheral endothelial dysfunction has been shown to be common in patients with coronary vasomotion abnormalities [107, 108].

6.6.2 Role of H₂O₂/EDH Factor in the Pathophysiology of Coronary Artery Disease

Previous studies focused on structural and functional abnormalities of "epicardial" coronary arteries in patients with CAD because they are easily visible on coronary angiography and amenable to procedural intervention (e.g. percutaneous coronary intervention). However, those of coronary microvasculature, referred to as CMD, have gained increasing attention as a novel research target in this population [12–14]. It is conceivable that impaired H_2O_2/EDH factor-mediated vasodilatation is involved in the pathogenesis of CMD in light of its potent vasodilator properties in coronary resistance vessels where EDH factors-mediated responses become relatively dominant to NO-mediated relaxations. A good example of this is that CMD caused by impaired H_2O_2/EDH factor is also associated with cardiac diastolic dysfunction in eNOS-KO mice [109]. Thus, it is essential to maintain the physiological balance between NO and H_2O_2/EDH factor for the treatment of CAD, which notion is supported by the fact that significant negative interactions exist between NO and several EDH factors [63, 88–91] and that nitrates as NO donors are not beneficial for the treatment of CMD [78, 80]. More recently, it has been highlighted that endothelium-dependent CMD is associated with low endothelial shear stress, larger plaque burden, and vulnerable plaque characteristic beyond conventional coronary risk factors in angina patients with INOCA [110, 111]. Shear stress is one of the important physiological cues that make endothelial cells synthesize and release EDRFs to maintain vascular homeostasis, while altered oscillatory or low shear stress with disturbed flow on coronary artery wall is implicated in the local progression of atherosclerotic coronary plaque through endothelial and VSMC proliferation, inflammation, lipoprotein uptake, and leukocyte adhesion [110, 111]. Indeed, altered shear stress on the coronary artery wall has been implicated in the local progression of atherosclerotic coronary plaque [112].

6.6.3 Lessons from Clinical Trials Targeting NO: Less Is More?

Although the role of CMD has been implicated in patients with obstructive CAD who underwent successful revascularization [113], the effects of isosorbide-5-mononitrate were unexpectedly neutral in patients with residual microvascular ischemia despite successful percutaneous coronary intervention [82]. Moreover, recent studies highlighted the high prevalence and pathophysiological relevance of CMD in patients with HFpEF [4–6]. Contrary to the premise that enhancing NO-mediated vasodilatation could exert beneficial effects on patients with HFpEF, the results of systemic and long-term administrations of inorganic nitrite in those patients were neutral or even harmful in randomized clinical trials [79, 81]. Similarly, antioxidant therapies for patients with cardiovascular diseases had no benefits [83], although multiple mechanisms may be involved in so-called "anti-oxidant paradox" in clinical trials, including inadequate dose, short treatment duration, and pro-oxidant effects of antioxidants upon supplementation. These lines of evidence indicate that it is important to turn our attention to avoid excessive NO supplementation and to pay attention to the potential harm of non-specific elimination of ROS by antioxidants. An alternative explanation for such "paradox" of NO-targeted therapy may be nitrosative stress induced by an excessive amount of supplemental NO [92, 114], again suggesting the importance of physiological balance between NO and EDH factors in endothelium-dependent vasodilatation. Although standard medications used for the treatment of cardiovascular diseases share the pleiotropic effects on endothelial function by enhancing NO-mediated vasodilatation with modest antioxidant capacities, including angiotensin-converting enzyme inhibitors, angiotensin II receptor blockers, and statins, further research is warranted to address how to modulate CMD to improve clinical outcomes of patients with cardiovascular diseases.

6.6.4 CMD as Systemic Vascular Dysfunction beyond the Heart

Recent studies have highlighted the importance of CMD with major clinical implications. First, if complicated with CMD, even angina patients who have angiographically normal coronary arteries or non-obstructive CAD are associated with increased future cardiac events, including myocardial infarction, percutaneous or surgical revascularization, cardiac death, and hospitalization for unstable angina [11, 12, 115, 116]. Moreover, the prevalence of CMD in this clinical entity is not negligible [8–11]. Although contemporary non-invasive stress tests have limited diagnostic accuracy for detecting CMD in patients with chest pain and non-obstructive CAD [9, 117], comprehensive invasive assessment of coronary vasomotor reactivity using intracoronary ACh, adenosine, and other vasoactive agents is safe, feasible, and of diagnostic value to identify patients with CMD [8, 9, 100, 104, 118]. Second, CMD is a cardiac manifestation of the systemic small artery disease [107], which supports the novel concept of "primary coronary microcirculatory dysfunction" [119]. Despite the high prevalence of CMD in patients with INOCA, they are often underestimated and offered no specific treatment or follow-up under the umbrella of "normal" coronary arteries. On the contrary to this otherwise common practice, patients with CMD are predisposed to future coronary events and associated worse outcomes [12, 115, 116]. Furthermore, CMD may be attributable to residual cardiac ischemia even after successful revascularization of significant epicardial coronary stenosis [113]. Identifying CMD in patients with stable IHD may provide physicians with useful information for decision making and risk stratification beyond conventional coronary risk factors.

6.7 Conclusions

This chapter highlighted the pathophysiology of CMD with emphasis placed on endothelial modulation of vascular tone mediated by H_2O_2/EDH factor and coronary microvascular spasm. It remains an open question for future research how to improve CMD without affecting the delicate balance between NO and EDH factors. Further characterization and better understanding of CMD are indispensable to this end, which helps us develop novel therapeutic strategies in patients with the disease.

Acknowledgments This work was supported in part by the Grants-in-Aid for Scientific Research from the Ministry of Education, Culture, Sports, Science and Technology, Tokyo, Japan, and the Grants-in-Aid for Scientific Research from the Ministry of Health, Labour, and Welfare, Tokyo, Japan.

References

1. Shimokawa H. 2014 Williams Harvey lecture: importance of coronary vasomotion abnormalities-from bench to bedside. Eur Heart J. 2014;35(45):3180–93. https://doi.org/10.1093/eurheartj/ehu427.
2. Kaski JC, Crea F, Gersh BJ, Camici PG. Reappraisal of ischemic heart disease. Circulation. 2018;138(14):1463–80. https://doi.org/10.1161/circulationaha.118.031373.
3. Michail M, Davies JE, Cameron JD, Parker KH, Brown AJ. Pathophysiological coronary and microcirculatory flow alterations in aortic stenosis. Nat Rev Cardiol. 2018;15(7):420–31. https://doi.org/10.1038/s41569-018-0011-2.
4. Crea F, Bairey Merz CN, Beltrame JF, Kaski JC, Ogawa H, Ong P, Sechtem U, Shimokawa H, Camici PG. The parallel tales of microvascular angina and heart failure with preserved ejection fraction: a paradigm shift. Eur Heart J. 2017;38(7):473–7. https://doi.org/10.1093/eurheartj/ehw461.
5. Dryer K, Gajjar M, Narang N, Lee M, Paul J, Shah AP, Nathan S, Butler J, Davidson CJ, Fearon WF, Shah SJ, Blair JEA. Coronary microvascular dysfunction in patients with heart failure with preserved ejection fraction. Am J Physiol Heart Circ Physiol. 2018;314(5):H1033–H42. https://doi.org/10.1152/ajpheart.00680.2017.
6. Shah SJ, Lam CSP, Svedlund S, Saraste A, Hage C, Tan RS, Beussink-Nelson L, Fermer ML, Broberg MA, Gan LM, Lund LH. Prevalence and correlates of coronary microvascular dysfunction in heart failure with preserved ejection fraction: PROMIS-HFpEF. Eur Heart J. 2018;39(37):3439–50. https://doi.org/10.1093/eurheartj/ehy531.
7. Patel MR, Peterson ED, Dai D, Brennan JM, Redberg RF, Anderson HV, Brindis RG, Douglas PS. Low diagnostic yield of elective coronary angiography. N Engl J Med. 2010;362(10):886–95. https://doi.org/10.1056/NEJMoa0907272.
8. Lee BK, Lim HS, Fearon WF, Yong AS, Yamada R, Tanaka S, Lee DP, Yeung AC, Tremmel JA. Invasive evaluation of patients with angina in the absence of obstructive coronary artery disease. Circulation. 2015;131(12):1054–60. https://doi.org/10.1161/circulationaha.114.012636.
9. Sara JD, Widmer RJ, Matsuzawa Y, Lennon RJ, Lerman LO, Lerman A. Prevalence of coronary microvascular dysfunction among patients with chest pain and nonobstructive coronary artery disease. J Am Coll Cardiol Intv. 2015;8(11):1445–53. https://doi.org/10.1016/j.jcin.2015.06.017.

10. Ford TJ, Yii E, Sidik N, Good R, Rocchiccioli P, McEntegart M, Watkins S, Eteiba H, Shaukat A, Lindsay M, Robertson K, Hood S, McGeoch R, McDade R, McCartney P, Corcoran D, Collison D, Rush C, Stanley B, McConnachie A, Sattar N, Touyz RM, Oldroyd KG, Berry C. Ischemia and no obstructive coronary artery disease: prevalence and correlates of coronary vasomotion disorders. Circ Cardiovasc Interv. 2019;12(12):e008126. https://doi.org/10.1161/circinterventions.119.008126.

11. Suda A, Takahashi J, Hao K, Kikuchi Y, Shindo T, Ikeda S, Sato K, Sugisawa J, Matsumoto Y, Miyata S, Sakata Y, Shimokawa H. Coronary functional abnormalities in patients with angina and nonobstructive coronary artery disease. J Am Coll Cardiol. 2019;74(19):2350–60. https://doi.org/10.1016/j.jacc.2019.08.1056.

12. Pepine CJ, Anderson RD, Sharaf BL, Reis SE, Smith KM, Handberg EM, Johnson BD, Sopko G, Bairey Merz CN. Coronary microvascular reactivity to adenosine predicts adverse outcome in women evaluated for suspected ischemia results from the National Heart, Lung and Blood Institute WISE (Women's ischemia syndrome evaluation) study. J Am Coll Cardiol. 2010;55(25):2825–32. https://doi.org/10.1016/j.jacc.2010.01.054.

13. Jespersen L, Hvelplund A, Abildstrom SZ, Pedersen F, Galatius S, Madsen JK, Jorgensen E, Kelbaek H, Prescott E. Stable angina pectoris with no obstructive coronary artery disease is associated with increased risks of major adverse cardiovascular events. Eur Heart J. 2012;33(6):734–44. https://doi.org/10.1093/eurheartj/ehr331.

14. Murthy VL, Naya M, Taqueti VR, Foster CR, Gaber M, Hainer J, Dorbala S, Blankstein R, Rimoldi O, Camici PG, Di Carli MF. Effects of sex on coronary microvascular dysfunction and cardiac outcomes. Circulation. 2014;129(24):2518–27. https://doi.org/10.1161/circulationaha.113.008507.

15. Camici PG, Crea F. Coronary microvascular dysfunction. N Engl J Med. 2007;356(8):830–40. https://doi.org/10.1056/NEJMra061889.

16. Crea F, Camici PG, Bairey Merz CN. Coronary microvascular dysfunction: an update. Eur Heart J. 2014;35(17):1101–11. https://doi.org/10.1093/eurheartj/eht513.

17. Crea F, Lanza G, Camici P. Mechanisms of coronary microvascular dysfunction. In: Coronary microvascular dysfunction. Milan: Springer; 2014. p. 31–47.

18. Camici PG, d'Amati G, Rimoldi O. Coronary microvascular dysfunction: mechanisms and functional assessment. Nat Rev Cardiol. 2015;12(1):48–62. https://doi.org/10.1038/nrcardio.2014.160.

19. Pries AR, Reglin B. Coronary microcirculatory pathophysiology: can we afford it to remain a black box? Eur Heart J. 2017;38(7):478–88. https://doi.org/10.1093/eurheartj/ehv760.

20. Shimokawa H. Reactive oxygen species in cardiovascular health and disease: special references to nitric oxide, hydrogen peroxide, and Rho-kinase. J Clin Biochem Nutr. 2020;66(2):83–91. https://doi.org/10.3164/jcbn.19-119.

21. Gould KL, Johnson NP. Coronary physiology beyond coronary flow reserve in microvascular angina: JACC state-of-the-art review. J Am Coll Cardiol. 2018;72(21):2642–62. https://doi.org/10.1016/j.jacc.2018.07.106.

22. Gutterman DD, Chabowski DS, Kadlec AO, Durand MJ, Freed JK, Ait-Aissa K, Beyer AM. The human microcirculation: regulation of flow and beyond. Circ Res. 2016;118(1):157–72. https://doi.org/10.1161/circresaha.115.305364.

23. Vanhoutte PM, Shimokawa H, Feletou M, Tang EH. Endothelial dysfunction and vascular disease -a 30th anniversary update. Acta Physiol. 2017;219(1):22–96. https://doi.org/10.1111/apha.12646.

24. Shimokawa H, Godo S. Nitric oxide and endothelium-dependent hyperpolarization mediated by hydrogen peroxide in health and disease. Basic Clin Pharmacol Toxicol. 2020;127(2):92–101. https://doi.org/10.1111/bcpt.13377.

25. Shimokawa H, Yasutake H, Fujii K, Owada MK, Nakaike R, Fukumoto Y, Takayanagi T, Nagao T, Egashira K, Fujishima M, Takeshita A. The importance of the hyperpolarizing mechanism increases as the vessel size decreases in endothelium-dependent relaxations in rat mesenteric circulation. J Cardiovasc Pharmacol. 1996;28(5):703–11. https://doi.org/10.1097/00005344-199611000-00014.

26. Urakami-Harasawa L, Shimokawa H, Nakashima M, Egashira K, Takeshita A. Importance of endothelium-derived hyperpolarizing factor in human arteries. J Clin Invest. 1997;100(11):2793–9. https://doi.org/10.1172/jci119826.

27. Ozkor MA, Murrow JR, Rahman AM, Kavtaradze N, Lin J, Manatunga A, Quyyumi AA. Endothelium-derived hyperpolarizing factor determines resting and stimulated forearm vasodilator tone in health and in disease. Circulation. 2011;123(20):2244–53. https://doi.org/10.1161/circulationaha.110.990317.

28. Vanhoutte PM. How we learned to say NO. Arterioscler Thromb Vasc Biol. 2009;29(8):1156–60. https://doi.org/10.1161/atvbaha.109.190215.

29. Feletou M, Kohler R, Vanhoutte PM. Nitric oxide: orchestrator of endothelium-dependent responses. Ann Med. 2012;44(7):694–716. https://doi.org/10.3109/07853890.2011.585658.

30. Vanhoutte PM, Zhao Y, Xu A, Leung SW. Thirty years of saying NO: sources, fate, actions, and misfortunes of the endothelium-derived vasodilator mediator. Circ Res. 2016;119(2):375–96. https://doi.org/10.1161/circresaha.116.306531.

31. Feletou M, Vanhoutte PM. Endothelium-dependent hyperpolarization of canine coronary smooth muscle. Br J Pharmacol. 1988;93(3):515–24. https://doi.org/10.1111/j.1476-5381.1988.tb10306.x.

32. Chen G, Suzuki H, Weston AH. Acetylcholine releases endothelium-derived hyperpolarizing factor and EDRF from rat blood vessels. Br J Pharmacol. 1988;95(4):1165–74. https://doi.org/10.1111/j.1476-5381.1988.tb11752.x.

33. Feletou M, Vanhoutte PM. EDHF: an update. Clin Sci. 2009;117(4):139–55. https://doi.org/10.1042/CS20090096.

34. Campbell WB, Gebremedhin D, Pratt PF, Harder DR. Identification of epoxyeicosatrienoic acids as endothelium-derived hyperpolarizing factors. Circ Res. 1996;78(3):415–23. https://doi.org/10.1161/01.res.78.3.415.

35. Fisslthaler B, Popp R, Kiss L, Potente M, Harder DR, Fleming I, Busse R. Cytochrome P450 2C is an EDHF synthase in coronary arteries. Nature. 1999;401(6752):493–7. https://doi.org/10.1038/46816.

36. Griffith TM, Chaytor AT, Edwards DH. The obligatory link: role of gap junctional communication in endothelium-dependent smooth muscle hyperpolarization. Pharmacol Res. 2004;49(6):551–64. https://doi.org/10.1016/j.phrs.2003.11.014.

37. Edwards G, Dora KA, Gardener MJ, Garland CJ, Weston AH. K+ is an endothelium-derived hyperpolarizing factor in rat arteries. Nature. 1998;396(6708):269–72. https://doi.org/10.1038/24388.

38. Matoba T, Shimokawa H, Nakashima M, Hirakawa Y, Mukai Y, Hirano K, Kanaide H, Takeshita A. Hydrogen peroxide is an endothelium-derived hyperpolarizing factor in mice. J Clin Invest. 2000;106(12):1521–30. https://doi.org/10.1172/jci10506.

39. Miura H, Gutterman DD. Human coronary arteriolar dilation to arachidonic acid depends on cytochrome P-450 monooxygenase and Ca^{2+}-activated K$^+$ channels. Circ Res. 1998;83(5):501–7. https://doi.org/10.1161/01.res.83.5.501.

40. Dora KA, Garland CJ. Properties of smooth muscle hyperpolarization and relaxation to K$^+$ in the rat isolated mesenteric artery. Am J Physiol Heart Circ Physiol. 2001;280(6):H2424–9. https://doi.org/10.1152/ajpheart.2001.280.6.H2424.

41. Beny JL, Schaad O. An evaluation of potassium ions as endothelium-derived hyperpolarizing factor in porcine coronary arteries. Br J Pharmacol. 2000;131(5):965–73. https://doi.org/10.1038/sj.bjp.0703658.

42. Nelli S, Wilson WS, Laidlaw H, Llano A, Middleton S, Price AG, Martin W. Evaluation of potassium ion as the endothelium-derived hyperpolarizing factor (EDHF) in the bovine coronary artery. Br J Pharmacol. 2003;139(5):982–8. https://doi.org/10.1038/sj.bjp.0705329.

43. Bussemaker E, Popp R, Binder J, Busse R, Fleming I. Characterization of the endothelium-derived hyperpolarizing factor (EDHF) response in the human interlobar artery. Kidney Int. 2003;63(5):1749–55. https://doi.org/10.1046/j.1523-1755.2003.00910.x.

44. Miura H, Bosnjak JJ, Ning G, Saito T, Miura M, Gutterman DD. Role for hydrogen peroxide in flow-induced dilation of human coronary arterioles. Circ Res. 2003;92(2):e31–40. https://doi.org/10.1161/01.res.0000054200.44505.ab.

45. Matoba T, Shimokawa H, Morikawa K, Kubota H, Kunihiro I, Urakami-Harasawa L, Mukai Y, Hirakawa Y, Akaike T, Takeshita A. Electron spin resonance detection of hydrogen peroxide as an endothelium-derived hyperpolarizing factor in porcine coronary microvessels. Arterioscler Thromb Vasc Biol. 2003;23(7):1224–30. https://doi.org/10.1161/01.atv.0000078601.79536.6c.

46. Yada T, Shimokawa H, Hiramatsu O, Kajita T, Shigeto F, Goto M, Ogasawara Y, Kajiya F. Hydrogen peroxide, an endogenous endothelium-derived hyperpolarizing factor, plays an important role in coronary autoregulation in vivo. Circulation. 2003;107(7):1040–5. https://doi.org/10.1161/01.cir.0000050145.25589.65.

47. Yada T, Shimokawa H, Hiramatsu O, Haruna Y, Morita Y, Kashihara N, Shinozaki Y, Mori H, Goto M, Ogasawara Y, Kajiya F. Cardioprotective role of endogenous hydrogen peroxide during ischemia-reperfusion injury in canine coronary microcirculation in vivo. Am J Physiol Heart Circ Physiol. 2006;291(3):H1138–46. https://doi.org/10.1152/ajpheart.00187.2006.

48. Yada T, Shimokawa H, Hiramatsu O, Shinozaki Y, Mori H, Goto M, Ogasawara Y, Kajiya F. Important role of endogenous hydrogen peroxide in pacing-induced metabolic coronary vasodilation in dogs in vivo. J Am Coll Cardiol. 2007;50(13):1272–8. https://doi.org/10.1016/j.jacc.2007.05.039.

49. Feletou M. The endothelium: part 2: EDHF-mediated responses "the classical pathway". San Rafael, CA: Morgan & Claypool Life Sciences Publisher; 2011.

50. Higashi Y, Sasaki S, Nakagawa K, Matsuura H, Oshima T, Chayama K. Endothelial function and oxidative stress in renovascular hypertension. N Engl J Med. 2002;346(25):1954–62. https://doi.org/10.1056/NEJMoa013591.

51. Holmstrom KM, Finkel T. Cellular mechanisms and physiological consequences of redox-dependent signalling. Nat Rev Mol Cell Biol. 2014;15(6):411–21. https://doi.org/10.1038/nrm3801.

52. Prysyazhna O, Rudyk O, Eaton P. Single atom substitution in mouse protein kinase G eliminates oxidant sensing to cause hypertension. Nat Med. 2012;18(2):286–90. https://doi.org/10.1038/nm.2603.

53. Nakajima S, Ohashi J, Sawada A, Noda K, Fukumoto Y, Shimokawa H. Essential role of bone marrow for microvascular endothelial and metabolic functions in mice. Circ Res. 2012;111(1):87–96. https://doi.org/10.1161/circresaha.112.270215.

54. Reddi AR, Culotta VC. SOD1 integrates signals from oxygen and glucose to repress respiration. Cell. 2013;152(1–2):224–35. https://doi.org/10.1016/j.cell.2012.11.046.

55. Rubanyi GM, Vanhoutte PM. Oxygen-derived free radicals, endothelium, and responsiveness of vascular smooth muscle. Am J Physiol. 1986;250:H815–21. https://doi.org/10.1152/ajpheart.1986.250.5.H815.

56. Nagao T, Illiano S, Vanhoutte PM. Calmodulin antagonists inhibit endothelium-dependent hyperpolarization in the canine coronary artery. Br J Pharmacol. 1992;107(2):382–6. https://doi.org/10.1111/j.1476-5381.1992.tb12755.x.

57. Matoba T, Shimokawa H, Kubota H, Morikawa K, Fujiki T, Kunihiro I, Mukai Y, Hirakawa Y, Takeshita A. Hydrogen peroxide is an endothelium-derived hyperpolarizing factor in human mesenteric arteries. Biochem Biophys Res Commun. 2002;290(3):909–13. https://doi.org/10.1006/bbrc.2001.6278.

58. Liu Y, Bubolz AH, Mendoza S, Zhang DX, Gutterman DD. H_2O_2 is the transferrable factor mediating flow-induced dilation in human coronary arterioles. Circ Res. 2011;108(5):566–73. https://doi.org/10.1161/circresaha.110.237636.

59. Lacza Z, Puskar M, Kis B, Perciaccante JV, Miller AW, Busija DW. Hydrogen peroxide acts as an EDHF in the piglet pial vasculature in response to bradykinin. Am J Physiol Heart Circ Physiol. 2002;283(1):H406–11. https://doi.org/10.1152/ajpheart.00007.2002.

60. Burgoyne JR, Oka S, Ale-Agha N, Eaton P. Hydrogen peroxide sensing and signaling by protein kinases in the cardiovascular system. Antioxid Redox Signal. 2013;18(9):1042–52. https://doi.org/10.1089/ars.2012.4817.

61. Zhang DX, Borbouse L, Gebremedhin D, Mendoza SA, Zinkevich NS, Li R, Gutterman DD. H_2O_2-induced dilation in human coronary arterioles: role of protein kinase G dimerization and large-conductance Ca^{2+}-activated K^+ channel activation. Circ Res. 2012;110(3):471–80. https://doi.org/10.1161/circresaha.111.258871.

62. Ohashi J, Sawada A, Nakajima S, Noda K, Takaki A, Shimokawa H. Mechanisms for enhanced endothelium-derived hyperpolarizing factor-mediated responses in microvessels in mice. Circ J. 2012;76(7):1768–79. https://doi.org/10.1253/circj.cj-12-0197.

63. Godo S, Sawada A, Saito H, Ikeda S, Enkhjargal B, Suzuki K, Tanaka S, Shimokawa H. Disruption of physiological balance between nitric oxide and endothelium-dependent hyperpolarization impairs cardiovascular homeostasis in mice. Arterioscler Thromb Vasc Biol. 2016;36(1):97–107. https://doi.org/10.1161/atvbaha.115.306499.

64. Garcia-Redondo AB, Briones AM, Beltran AE, Alonso MJ, Simonsen U, Salaices M. Hypertension increases contractile responses to hydrogen peroxide in resistance arteries through increased thromboxane A_2, Ca^{2+}, and superoxide anion levels. J Pharmacol Exp Ther. 2009;328(1):19–27. https://doi.org/10.1124/jpet.108.144295.

65. Antunes F, Cadenas E. Estimation of H_2O_2 gradients across biomembranes. FEBS Lett. 2000;475(2):121–6. https://doi.org/10.1016/s0014-5793(00)01638-0.

66. Takaki A, Morikawa K, Murayama Y, Yamagishi H, Hosoya M, Ohashi J, Shimokawa H. Roles of endothelial oxidases in endothelium-derived hyperpolarizing factor responses in mice. J Cardiovasc Pharmacol. 2008;52(6):510–7. https://doi.org/10.1097/FJC.0b013e318190358b.

67. Morikawa K, Shimokawa H, Matoba T, Kubota H, Akaike T, Talukder MA, Hatanaka M, Fujiki T, Maeda H, Takahashi S, Takeshita A. Pivotal role of Cu,Zn-superoxide dismutase in endothelium-dependent hyperpolarization. J Clin Invest. 2003;112(12):1871–9. https://doi.org/10.1172/jci19351.

68. Liu Y, Zhao H, Li H, Kalyanaraman B, Nicolosi AC, Gutterman DD. Mitochondrial sources of H_2O_2 generation play a key role in flow-mediated dilation in human coronary resistance arteries. Circ Res. 2003;93(6):573–80. https://doi.org/10.1161/01.res.0000091261.19387.ae.

69. Larsen BT, Bubolz AH, Mendoza SA, Pritchard KA Jr, Gutterman DD. Bradykinin-induced dilation of human coronary arterioles requires NADPH oxidase-derived reactive oxygen species. Arterioscler Thromb Vasc Biol. 2009;29(5):739–45. https://doi.org/10.1161/atvbaha.108.169367.

70. Sartoretto JL, Kalwa H, Pluth MD, Lippard SJ, Michel T. Hydrogen peroxide differentially modulates cardiac myocyte nitric oxide synthesis. Proc Natl Acad Sci U S A. 2011;108(38):15792–7. https://doi.org/10.1073/pnas.1111331108.

71. Shiroto T, Romero N, Sugiyama T, Sartoretto JL, Kalwa H, Yan Z, Shimokawa H, Michel T. Caveolin-1 is a critical determinant of autophagy, metabolic switching, and oxidative stress in vascular endothelium. PLoS One. 2014;9(2):e87871. https://doi.org/10.1371/journal.pone.0087871.

72. Freed JK, Beyer AM, LoGiudice JA, Hockenberry JC, Gutterman DD. Ceramide changes the mediator of flow-induced vasodilation from nitric oxide to hydrogen peroxide in the human microcirculation. Circ Res. 2014;115(5):525–32. https://doi.org/10.1161/circresaha.115.303881.

73. Beyer AM, Freed JK, Durand MJ, Riedel M, Ait-Aissa K, Green P, Hockenberry JC, Morgan RG, Donato AJ, Peleg R, Gasparri M, Rokkas CK, Santos JH, Priel E, Gutterman DD. Critical role for telomerase in the mechanism of flow-mediated dilation in the human microcirculation. Circ Res. 2016;118(5):856–66. https://doi.org/10.1161/circresaha.115.307918.

74. Shimokawa H. Hydrogen peroxide as an endothelium-derived hyperpolarizing factor. Pflugers Arch. 2010;459(6):915–22. https://doi.org/10.1007/s00424-010-0790-8.

75. Chidgey J, Fraser PA, Aaronson PI. Reactive oxygen species facilitate the EDH response in arterioles by potentiating intracellular endothelial Ca^{2+} release. Free Radic Biol Med. 2016;97:274–84. https://doi.org/10.1016/j.freeradbiomed.2016.06.010.
76. Burgoyne JR, Madhani M, Cuello F, Charles RL, Brennan JP, Schroder E, Browning DD, Eaton P. Cysteine redox sensor in $PKGI\alpha$ enables oxidant-induced activation. Science. 2007;317(5843):1393–7. https://doi.org/10.1126/science.1144318.
77. Dou D, Zheng X, Liu J, Xu X, Ye L, Gao Y. Hydrogen peroxide enhances vasodilatation by increasing dimerization of cGMP-dependent protein kinase type Iα. Circ J. 2012;76(7):1792–8. https://doi.org/10.1253/circj.cj-11-1368.
78. Russo G, Di Franco A, Lamendola P, Tarzia P, Nerla R, Stazi A, Villano A, Sestito A, Lanza GA, Crea F. Lack of effect of nitrates on exercise stress test results in patients with microvascular angina. Cardiovasc Drugs Ther. 2013;27(3):229–34. https://doi.org/10.1007/s10557-013-6439-z.
79. Redfield MM, Anstrom KJ, Levine JA, Koepp GA, Borlaug BA, Chen HH, LeWinter MM, Joseph SM, Shah SJ, Semigran MJ, Felker GM, Cole RT, Reeves GR, Tedford RJ, Tang WH, McNulty SE, Velazquez EJ, Shah MR, Braunwald E. Isosorbide mononitrate in heart failure with preserved ejection fraction. N Engl J Med. 2015;373(24):2314–24. https://doi.org/10.1056/NEJMoa1510774.
80. Takahashi J, Nihei T, Takagi Y, Miyata S, Odaka Y, Tsunoda R, Seki A, Sumiyoshi T, Matsui M, Goto T, Tanabe Y, Sueda S, Momomura SI, Yasuda S, Ogawa H, Shimokawa H. Prognostic impact of chronic nitrate therapy in patients with vasospastic angina: multicentre registry study of the Japanese coronary spasm association. Eur Heart J. 2015;36(4):228–37. https://doi.org/10.1093/eurheartj/ehu313.
81. Borlaug BA, Anstrom KJ, Lewis GD, Shah SJ, Levine JA, Koepp GA, Givertz MM, Felker GM, LeWinter MM, Mann DL, Margulies KB, Smith AL, Tang WHW, Whellan DJ, Chen HH, Davila-Roman VG, McNulty S, Desvigne-Nickens P, Hernandez AF, Braunwald E, Redfield MM. Effect of inorganic nitrite vs placebo on exercise capacity among patients with heart failure with preserved ejection fraction: the INDIE-HFpEF randomized clinical trial. JAMA. 2018;320(17):1764–73. https://doi.org/10.1001/jama.2018.14852.
82. Golino M, Spera FR, Manfredonia L, De Vita A, Di Franco A, Lamendola P, Villano A, Melita V, Mencarelli E, Lanza GA, Crea F. Microvascular ischemia in patients with successful percutaneous coronary intervention: effects of ranolazine and isosorbide-5-mononitrate. Eur Rev Med Pharmacol Sci. 2018;22(19):6545–50. https://doi.org/10.26355/eurrev_201810_16070.
83. Bjelakovic G, Nikolova D, Gluud LL, Simonetti RG, Gluud C. Mortality in randomized trials of antioxidant supplements for primary and secondary prevention: systematic review and meta-analysis. JAMA. 2007;297(8):842–57. https://doi.org/10.1001/jama.297.8.842.
84. Takaki A, Morikawa K, Tsutsui M, Murayama Y, Tekes E, Yamagishi H, Ohashi J, Yada T, Yanagihara N, Shimokawa H. J Exp Med. 2008;205(9):2053–63. https://doi.org/10.1084/jem.20080106.
85. Forstermann U, Li H. Therapeutic effect of enhancing endothelial nitric oxide synthase (eNOS) expression and preventing eNOS uncoupling. Br J Pharmacol. 2011;164(2):213–23. https://doi.org/10.1111/j.1476-5381.2010.01196.x.
86. Stuehr D, Pou S, Rosen GM. Oxygen reduction by nitric-oxide synthases. J Biol Chem. 2001;276(18):14533–6. https://doi.org/10.1074/jbc.R100011200.
87. Huang PL, Huang Z, Mashimo H, Bloch KD, Moskowitz MA, Bevan JA, Fishman MC. Hypertension in mice lacking the gene for endothelial nitric oxide synthase. Nature. 1995;377(6546):239–42. https://doi.org/10.1038/377239a0.
88. Bauersachs J, Popp R, Hecker M, Sauer E, Fleming I, Busse R. Nitric oxide attenuates the release of endothelium-derived hyperpolarizing factor. Circulation. 1996;94(12):3341–7. https://doi.org/10.1161/01.cir.94.12.3341.
89. Nishikawa Y, Stepp DW, Chilian WM. Nitric oxide exerts feedback inhibition on EDHF-induced coronary arteriolar dilation in vivo. Am J Physiol Heart Circ Physiol. 2000;279(2):H459–65. https://doi.org/10.1152/ajpheart.2000.279.2.H459.

90. Olmos L, Mombouli JV, Illiano S, Vanhoutte PM. cGMP mediates the desensitization to bradykinin in isolated canine coronary arteries. Am J Physiol. 1995;268(2 Pt 2):H865–70. https://doi.org/10.1152/ajpheart.1995.268.2.H865.

91. Burgoyne JR, Prysyazhna O, Rudyk O, Eaton P. cGMP-dependent activation of protein kinase G precludes disulfide activation: implications for blood pressure control. Hypertension. 2012;60(5):1301–8. https://doi.org/10.1161/hypertensionaha.112.198754.

92. Saito H, Godo S, Sato S, Ito A, Ikumi Y, Tanaka S, Ida T, Fujii S, Akaike T, Shimokawa H. Important role of endothelial caveolin-1 in the protective role of endothelium-dependent hyperpolarization against nitric oxide-mediated nitrative stress in microcirculation in mice. J Cardiovasc Pharmacol. 2018;71(2):113–26. https://doi.org/10.1097/fjc.0000000000000552.

93. Enkhjargal B, Godo S, Sawada A, Suvd N, Saito H, Noda K, Satoh K, Shimokawa H. Endothelial AMP-activated protein kinase regulates blood pressure and coronary flow responses through hyperpolarization mechanism in mice. Arterioscler Thromb Vasc Biol. 2014;34:1505–13. https://doi.org/10.1161/atvbaha.114.303735.

94. Kikuchi Y, Yasuda S, Aizawa K, Tsuburaya R, Ito Y, Takeda M, Nakayama M, Ito K, Takahashi J, Shimokawa H. Enhanced Rho-kinase activity in circulating neutrophils of patients with vasospastic angina: a possible biomarker for diagnosis and disease activity assessment. J Am Coll Cardiol. 2011;58(12):1231–7. https://doi.org/10.1016/j.jacc.2011.05.046.

95. Nihei T, Takahashi J, Hao K, Kikuchi Y, Odaka Y, Tsuburaya R, Nishimiya K, Matsumoto Y, Ito K, Miyata S, Sakata Y, Shimokawa H. Prognostic impacts of Rho-kinase activity in circulating leucocytes in patients with vasospastic angina. Eur Heart J. 2018;39(11):952–9. https://doi.org/10.1093/eurheartj/ehx657.

96. Mohri M, Shimokawa H, Hirakawa Y, Masumoto A, Takeshita A. Rho-kinase inhibition with intracoronary fasudil prevents myocardial ischemia in patients with coronary microvascular spasm. J Am Coll Cardiol. 2003;41(1):15–9. https://doi.org/10.1016/s0735-1097(02)02632-3.

97. Kikuchi Y, Takahashi J, Hao K, Sato K, Sugisawa J, Tsuchiya S, Suda A, Shindo T, Ikeda S, Shiroto T, Matsumoto Y, Miyata S, Sakata Y, Shimokawa H. Usefulness of intracoronary administration of fasudil, a selective Rho-kinase inhibitor, for PCI-related refractory myocardial ischemia. Int J Cardiol. 2019;297:8–13. https://doi.org/10.1016/j.ijcard.2019.09.057.

98. Halcox JP, Nour KR, Zalos G, Quyyumi AA. Endogenous endothelin in human coronary vascular function: differential contribution of endothelin receptor types A and B. Hypertension. 2007;49(5):1134–41. https://doi.org/10.1161/hypertensionaha.106.083303.

99. Odaka Y, Takahashi J, Tsuburaya R, Nishimiya K, Hao K, Matsumoto Y, Ito K, Sakata Y, Miyata S, Manita D, Hirowatari Y, Shimokawa H. Plasma concentration of serotonin is a novel biomarker for coronary microvascular dysfunction in patients with suspected angina and unobstructive coronary arteries. Eur Heart J. 2017;38(7):489–96. https://doi.org/10.1093/eurheartj/ehw448.

100. Lanza GA. Diagnostic approach to patients with stable angina and no obstructive coronary arteries. Eur Cardiol. 2019;14(2):97–102. https://doi.org/10.15420/ecr.2019.22.2.

101. Mohri M, Koyanagi M, Egashira K, Tagawa H, Ichiki T, Shimokawa H, Takeshita A. Angina pectoris caused by coronary microvascular spasm. Lancet. 1998;351(9110):1165–9. https://doi.org/10.1016/s0140-6736(97)07329-7.

102. Ong P, Athanasiadis A, Borgulya G, Mahrholdt H, Kaski JC, Sechtem U. High prevalence of a pathological response to acetylcholine testing in patients with stable angina pectoris and unobstructed coronary arteries. The ACOVA study (Abnormal COronary VAsomotion in patients with stable angina and unobstructed coronary arteries). J Am Coll Cardiol. 2012;59(7):655–62. https://doi.org/10.1016/j.jacc.2011.11.015.

103. Ong P, Camici PG, Beltrame JF, Crea F, Shimokawa H, Sechtem U, Kaski JC, Bairey Merz CN. International standardization of diagnostic criteria for microvascular angina. Int J Cardiol. 2018;250:16–20. https://doi.org/10.1016/j.ijcard.2017.08.068.

104. Ford TJ, Stanley B, Good R, Rocchiccioli P, McEntegart M, Watkins S, Eteiba H, Shaukat A, Lindsay M, Robertson K, Hood S, McGeoch R, McDade R, Yii E, Sidik N, McCartney P, Corcoran D, Collison D, Rush C, McConnachie A, Touyz RM, Oldroyd KG, Berry

C. Stratified medical therapy using invasive coronary function testing in angina: the CorMicA trial. J Am Coll Cardiol. 2018;72(23):2841–55. https://doi.org/10.1016/j.jacc.2018.09.006.

105. Matsuzawa Y, Kwon TG, Lennon RJ, Lerman LO, Lerman A. Prognostic value of flow-mediated vasodilation in brachial artery and fingertip artery for cardiovascular events: a systematic review and meta-analysis. J Am Heart Assoc. 2015;4(11):e002270. https://doi.org/10.1161/jaha.115.002270.

106. Chadderdon SM, Belcik JT, Bader L, Peters DM, Kievit P, Alkayed NJ, Kaul S, Grove KL, Lindner JR. Temporal changes in skeletal muscle capillary responses and endothelial-derived vasodilators in obesity-related insulin resistance. Diabetes. 2016;65(8):2249–57. https://doi.org/10.2337/db15-1574.

107. Ford TJ, Rocchiccioli P, Good R, McEntegart M, Eteiba H, Watkins S, Shaukat A, Lindsay M, Robertson K, Hood S, Yii E, Sidik N, Harvey A, Montezano AC, Beattie E, Haddow L, Oldroyd KG, Touyz RM, Berry C. Systemic microvascular dysfunction in microvascular and vasospastic angina. Eur Heart J. 2018;39(46):4086–97. https://doi.org/10.1093/eurheartj/ehy529.

108. Ohura-Kajitani S, Shiroto T, Godo S, Ikumi Y, Ito A, Tanaka S, Sato K, Sugisawa J, Tsuchiya S, Suda A, Shindo T, Ikeda S, Hao K, Kikuchi Y, Nochioka K, Matsumoto Y, Takahashi J, Miyata S, Shimokawa H. Marked impairment of endothelium-dependent digital vasodilatations in patients with microvascular angina: evidence for systemic small artery disease. Arterioscler Thromb Vasc Biol. 2020;40(5):1400–12. https://doi.org/10.1161/atvbaha.119.313704.

109. Ikumi Y, Shiroto T, Godo S, Saito H, Tanaka S, Ito A, Kajitani S, Monma Y, Miyata S, Tsutsui M, Shimokawa H. Important roles of endothelium-dependent hyperpolarization in coronary microcirculation and cardiac diastolic function in mice. J Cardiovasc Pharmacol. 2020;75(1):31–40. https://doi.org/10.1097/fjc.0000000000000763.

110. Siasos G, Sara JD, Zaromytidou M, Park KH, Coskun AU, Lerman LO, Oikonomou E, Maynard CC, Fotiadis D, Stefanou K, Papafaklis M, Michalis L, Feldman C, Lerman A, Stone PH. Local low shear stress and endothelial dysfunction in patients with nonobstructive coronary atherosclerosis. J Am Coll Cardiol. 2018;71(19):2092–102. https://doi.org/10.1016/j.jacc.2018.02.073.

111. Godo S, Corban MT, Toya T, Gulati R, Lerman LO, Lerman A. Association of coronary microvascular endothelial dysfunction with vulnerable plaque characteristics in early coronary atherosclerosis. EuroIntervention. (in press). 2019; https://doi.org/10.4244/eij-d-19-00265.

112. Corban MT, Eshtehardi P, Suo J, McDaniel MC, Timmins LH, Rassoul-Arzrumly E, Maynard C, Mekonnen G, King S 3rd, Quyyumi AA, Giddens DP, Samady H. Combination of plaque burden, wall shear stress, and plaque phenotype has incremental value for prediction of coronary atherosclerotic plaque progression and vulnerability. Atherosclerosis. 2014;232(2):271–6. https://doi.org/10.1016/j.atherosclerosis.2013.11.049.

113. Al-Lamee R, Thompson D, Dehbi HM, Sen S, Tang K, Davies J, Keeble T, Mielewczik M, Kaprielian R, Malik IS, Nijjer SS, Petraco R, Cook C, Ahmad Y, Howard J, Baker C, Sharp A, Gerber R, Talwar S, Assomull R, Mayet J, Wensel R, Collier D, Shun-Shin M, Thom SA, Davies JE, Francis DP. Percutaneous coronary intervention in stable angina (ORBITA): a double-blind, randomised controlled trial. Lancet. 2018;391(10115):31–40. https://doi.org/10.1016/s0140-6736(17)32714-9.

114. Schiattarella GG, Altamirano F, Tong D, French KM, Villalobos E, Kim SY, Luo X, Jiang N, May HI, Wang ZV, Hill TM, Mammen PPA, Huang J, Lee DI, Hahn VS, Sharma K, Kass DA, Lavandero S, Gillette TG, Hill JA. Nitrosative stress drives heart failure with preserved ejection fraction. Nature. 2019;568(7752):351–6. https://doi.org/10.1038/s41586-019-1100-z.

115. Suwaidi JA, Hamasaki S, Higano ST, Nishimura RA, Holmes DR Jr, Lerman A. Long-term follow-up of patients with mild coronary artery disease and endothelial dysfunction. Circulation. 2000;101(9):948–54. https://doi.org/10.1161/01.CIR.101.9.948.

116. Halcox JP, Schenke WH, Zalos G, Mincemoyer R, Prasad A, Waclawiw MA, Nour KR, Quyyumi AA. Prognostic value of coronary vascular endothelial dysfunction. Circulation. 2002;106(6):653–8. https://doi.org/10.1161/01.cir.0000025404.78001.d8.

117. Cassar A, Chareonthaitawee P, Rihal CS, Prasad A, Lennon RJ, Lerman LO, Lerman A. Lack of correlation between noninvasive stress tests and invasive coronary vasomotor dysfunction in patients with nonobstructive coronary artery disease. Circ Cardiovasc Interv. 2009;2(3):237–44. https://doi.org/10.1161/circinterventions.108.841056.

118. Ong P, Athanasiadis A, Borgulya G, Vokshi I, Bastiaenen R, Kubik S, Hill S, Schaufele T, Mahrholdt H, Kaski JC, Sechtem U. Clinical usefulness, angiographic characteristics, and safety evaluation of intracoronary acetylcholine provocation testing among 921 consecutive white patients with unobstructed coronary arteries. Circulation. 2014;129(17):1723–30. https://doi.org/10.1161/circulationaha.113.004096.

119. Lerman A, Holmes DR, Herrmann J, Gersh BJ. Microcirculatory dysfunction in ST-elevation myocardial infarction: cause, consequence, or both? Eur Heart J. 2007;28(7):788–97. https://doi.org/10.1093/eurheartj/ehl501.

Chapter 7
Diagnosis of Coronary Microvascular Dysfunction

Jun Takahashi and Hiroaki Shimokawa

Abstract Coronary microvascular dysfunction (CMD) has emerged as a third potential mechanism of myocardial ischemia in addition to coronary atherosclerotic disease (CAD) and epicardial coronary artery spasm. Since several studies indicated that CMD could be associated with increased risk of cardiovascular events, it is important to make correct diagnosis and assessment of CMD. However, in contrast with epicardial coronary arteries, the coronary microcirculation cannot be directly visualized in vivo with coronary angiography or intracoronary imaging technique. Although there are several non-invasive (e.g. transthoracic Doppler echocardiography, positron emission tomography, cardiac magnetic resonance imaging) and invasive (e.g. assessment of coronary flow reserve and microvascular resistance using adenosine, microvascular coronary spasm with acetylcholine) approaches for the evaluation of coronary microvascular function, all of them have several limitations. Currently, the interventional diagnostic procedure, which consists of acetylcholine testing for the detection of coronary spasm as well as coronary flow reserve and microvascular resistance assessment in response to adenosine using a coronary pressure–temperature sensor guidewire, could represent the most comprehensive coronary vasomotor evaluation. Furthermore, several biomarkers have recently attracted much attention as a diagnostic tool for CMD. Especially, plasma concentration of serotonin may be a novel biomarker to dissect CMD from epicardial coronary artery spasm. Correct diagnosis of the underlying cause of angina should enable us to stratify the treatment for distinct disorders, including CMD, vasospastic angina, and non-cardiac chest pain.

Keywords Non-invasive approach · Coronary vasoreactivity testing · Coronary flow reserve · Coronary microvascular resistance · Microvascular spasm · Biomarker

J. Takahashi · H. Shimokawa (✉)
Department of Cardiovascular Medicine, Tohoku University Graduate School of Medicine, Sendai, Miyagi, Japan
e-mail: shimo@cardio.med.tohoku.ac.jp

© Springer Nature Singapore Pte Ltd. 2021
H. Shimokawa (ed.), *Coronary Vasomotion Abnormalities*,
https://doi.org/10.1007/978-981-15-7594-5_7

7.1 Introduction

It has been reported that up to 40% of patients undergoing diagnostic coronary angiography for typical chest pain have no significant coronary stenosis [1]. The Women's Ischemia Syndrome Evaluation Study showed that there are at least 3–4 million patients in the United States alone who have signs and symptoms of myocardial ischemia with non-obstructive coronary artery disease (CAD), associated with poor quality of life, psychological distress, and health-care costs that approximate those of patients with obstructive CAD [2, 3]. In such cases, myocardial ischemia may be caused by different types of functional disorders involving the epicardial coronary arteries, coronary microcirculation or both [4]. Vasospastic angina (VSA) is one of the important functional cardiac disorders characterized by myocardial ischemia attributable to epicardial coronary artery spasm and a number of studies have elucidated patient characteristics, outcomes, and prognostic factors of VSA [5–7]. Furthermore, the Japanese Circulation Society guidelines describe the standard methods for the diagnosis of VSA in the current clinical practice based on the currently available evidence [8]. The Coronary Vasomotion Disorders International Study Group (COVADIS) also developed international standards for the diagnostic criteria of VSA [9]. Remarkably, the spasm provocation tests with ergonovine and acetylcholine employed in the catheterization laboratory have been established as a high-reliable diagnostic tool to detect functional disorder of the epicardial coronary artery [10, 11]. We also have recently demonstrated that Rho-kinase activity in circulating neutrophils is enhanced in VSA patients and is a useful biomarker for diagnosis and disease activity assessment of the disorder [12, 13]. On the other hand, coronary microvascular dysfunction (CMD) has emerged as a third potential mechanism of myocardial ischemia in addition to coronary atherosclerotic disease and epicardial coronary spasm [4, 14]. Indeed, it was demonstrated that CMD could be associated with increased risk of cardiovascular events, [15] indicating that it is important to make a correct diagnosis or assessment of CMD. However, in contrast with epicardial coronary arteries, the coronary microcirculation cannot be directly visualized in vivo with coronary angiography or intracoronary imaging technique. Thus, microvascular function is assessed indirectly, generally through measurements of coronary or myocardial blood flow (MBF) which is regulated by coronary arteriolar tone in healthy vessels, or detection of propensity to coronary vasoconstriction. A number of studies published in the past 2 decades have highlighted how abnormalities in the function and structure of the coronary microcirculation can interfere with the control of MBF, and contribute to the pathogenesis of myocardial ischemia [16]. In this chapter, we will briefly review the diagnostic methods and strategies for CMD.

7.2   Clinical Criteria for Suspecting Microvascular Angina Due to CMD

CMD could be developed by several pathological mechanisms. In 2007, Camici and Crea proposed the clinical and pathogenetic classifications of CMD (Table 7.1) [14]. From a pathophysiological point of view, and independently of the underlying mechanisms, CMD results in varying degrees of disruption of the normal coronary physiology. These alterations eventually impair the capacity of MBF to adapt to changes in myocardial oxygen demand. Indeed, CMD is typically suspected in patients with angina and nearly normal coronary angiograms. The term "microvascular angina" (MVA) typically describes myocardial ischemia triggered by CMD in the absence of CAD. Stable MVA is characterized by effort-induced symptoms similar to those observed in patients with angina triggered by obstructive CAD. However, MVA patients often have angina at rest and a variable angina threshold, suggestive of dynamic coronary vasomotor changes. CMD can result from a variable combination of abnormal vasodilatation and increased vasoconstriction caused by various stimuli of coronary microvessels (Fig. 7.1) [17]. Thus, the presence of both effort and rest angina suggests a possible coexistence of reduced coronary microvascular dilatory function and microvascular spasm [18]. Patients

Table 7.1 Classification of coronary microvascular dysfunction

	Clinical setting	Main pathogenic mechanism
Type 1: in the absence of myocardial diseases and obstructive CAD	Risk factors	SMC dysfunction
	Microvascular angina	Endothelial dysfunction
		Vascular remodeling
Type 2: in myocardial diseases	Hypertrophic cardiomyopathy	Vascular remodeling
	Dilated cardiomyopathy	SMC dysfunction
	Anderson-Fabry's disease	Extramural compression
	Amyloidosis	Luminal obstruction
	Myocarditis	
	Aortic stenosis	
Type 3: obstructive CAD	Stable angina	SMC dysfunction
	Acute coronary syndrome	Endothelial dysfunction
		Luminal obstruction
Type 4: iatrogenic	PCI	Luminal obstruction
	Coronary artery grafting	Autonomic dysfunction

CAD coronary artery disease, *SMC* smooth muscle cells, *PCI* percutaneous coronary intervention. (Reproduced from Crea et al. [14])

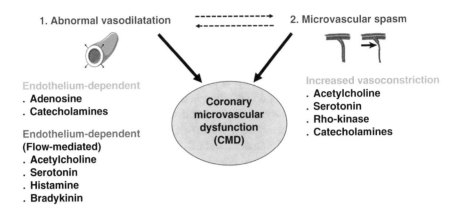

Fig. 7.1 Coronary microvascular dysfunction car result from a variable combination of abnormal vasodilatation and increased vasoconstriction caused by various stimuli

with MVA may have chest pain that can persist even after cessation of the activity [19]. Furthermore, they may not have rapid or sufficient symptom relief in response to sublingual nitroglycerin, because nitroglycerin selectively dilates larger microvessels but not arterioles [20]. Furthermore, typical and atypical chest pain does not differentiate between obstructive and non-obstructive CAD and symptom complexity may not always identify patients with CMD [21, 22]. Excluding angiographic atheroma or establishing that a stenosis has no effect on coronary physiology (e.g. normal fractional flow reserve) strongly suggests a microvascular origin of symptoms [23]. Although objective documentation of myocardial ischemia is warranted for the diagnosis of CMD, imaging modalities often give negative results despite the occurrence of ischemia. This is because, contrary to what is seen in obstructive CAD, myocardial ischemia does not follow a regional pattern in MVA and ischemia may be limited to the subendocardium in many cases [19]. Based on these clinical features of MVA, the Coronary Vasomotor Disorder Study (COVADIS) group has recently proposed the following diagnostic criteria for MVA [24]; signs and symptoms of myocardial ischemia, reduced coronary flow reserve (CFR) defined as the ratio of coronary blood flow (CBF) during near maximal coronary vasodilatation to baseline CBF, or microvascular spasm, and documented myocardial ischemia, which is not triggered by obstructive CAD but by functional or structural abnormalities at the site of the coronary microcirculation (Table 7.2). Angina occurs in approximately 30–60% of patients with CMD [22, 25–28]. Other cardinal manifestations of CMD include exertional dyspnea and possibly heart failure [29]. Patients may also manifest with a gradual decrease in exercise tolerance or dyspnea on exertion. It may represent an ischemic equivalent caused by LV diastolic dysfunction with an excessive rise in end-diastolic pressure leading to cardiopulmonary congestion. In those patients presenting with heart failure, the typical signs of elevated filling pressure, such as jugular venous distention, rales, and pedal edema, may be present.

Table 7.2 Clinical criteria for suspecting microvascular angina

1.	Symptoms of myocardial ischemia
	(a) Effort and/or rest angina
	(b) Angina equivalents (e.g. shortness of breath)
2.	Absence of obstructive CAD (<50% diameter reduction or FFR > 0.80) by
	(a) Coronary CTA
	(b) Invasive coronary angiography
3.	Objective evidence of myocardial ischemia
	(a) Ischemic ECG changes during an episode of chest pain
	(b) Stress-induced chest pain and/or ischemic ECG changes in the presence or absence of transient/reversible abnormal myocardial perfusion and/or wall motion abnormality
4.	Evidence of impaired coronary microvascular function
	(a) Impaired coronary flow reserve (cut-off values depending on methodology use between ≤2.0 and ≤ 2.5)
	(b) Coronary microvascular spasm, defined as reproduction of symptoms, ischemic ECG shifts but no epicardial spasm during acetylcholine testing
	(c) Abnormal coronary microvascular resistance indices (e.g. IMR > 25)
	(d) Coronary slow flow phenomenon, defined as TIMI frame count >25
	CAD coronary artery disease, *CTA* computed tomographic angiography, *FFR* fractional flow reserve, *IMR* index of microcirculatory resistance, *TIMI* thrombolysis in myocardial infarction
	Definite MVA is only diagnosed if all four criteria are present
	Suspected MVA is diagnosed if symptoms of ischemia are present with non-obstructive
	CAD but only objective evidence of myocardial ischemia, or evidence of impaired coronary microvascular function alone

(Reproduced from Ong et al. [24])

7.3 Assessment for Diastolic Function of Coronary Microvasculature

Coronary microvascular function is usually assessed by measurement of coronary microvascular response to vasodilator stimuli. In many cases, the vasodilator capacity is often evaluated by CFR calculated as the ratio of CBF during maximal vasodilatation over basal CBF. Since CFR is an integrated measure of flow through both the large epicardial arteries and the coronary microcirculation, reduced CFR is a marker of CMD in the absence of obstructive stenosis of the epicardial arteries [16]. The most widely used substance to assess coronary microvascular dilator function is adenosine. Adenosine is administered at an intravenous dose of 140 μg/kg/min, as this dose has been found to achieve maximal coronary microvascular dilatation [30]. Although adenosine has possible side effects, including bradycardia due to atrioventricular or sino-atrial node blockade and bronchoconstriction, both of which are mediated by purinergic A1 receptor, relevant advantages of adenosine are its very short half-life (10 s) which enables rapid regression of side effects and repetition of the test during the same session, if necessary [31]. Another frequently used substance to assess endothelium-independent coronary microvascular dilatation is dipyridamole, which acts by inhibiting adenosine degradation by adenosine deaminase [32]. Acetylcholine is often used as a endothelium-dependent coronary microvascular vasodilator. However, it is not the ideal substance to assess endothelium-dependent vasodilator function, since it also acts directly on smooth muscle cells (SMCs), including vasoconstriction [4]. There are several non-invasive and invasive approaches for evaluation of coronary vasodilator response, while all of them have several limitations. Although there is currently no consensus on the cut-off for the diagnosis of CMD based on imaging, a three-tiered characterization of CMD has been proposed as follows: CFR < 1.5, definite; CMD 1.5–2.6, borderline; and CMD >2.6, no CMD [33].

7.3.1 Non-invasive Techniques for Diagnosis of CMD

Transthoracic Doppler echocardiography (TTDE) can measure coronary blood flow velocity (CBFV) of the distal left anterior descending artery (LAD), which is a surrogate for CBF. CFR is measured as the ratio of peak CBFV after vasodilator to CBFV at rest in a highly reproducible fashion [34]. CFR measured by TTDE has been demonstrated to have good agreement with that measured by an intracoronary Doppler flow wire and positron emission tomography (PET) [34, 35]. Advantages of TTDE are its relatively low cost and high feasibility, but considerable intra-observer and inter-observer variability (~10%) needs to be taken into account when examining serial recordings obtained for assessing the effects of therapy [36]. Myocardial contrast echocardiography (MCE) exploits the property of intravenously administered, echogenic, gas-filled microbubbles that are similar in size and rheological properties to red blood cells [37]. MCE enables repeated, quantitative measurement of microvascular flow velocity and capillary blood volume, and provides an estimate of MBF that correlated well with that measured by PET [38]. There is a growing body of evidence that a reduced coronary flow velocity reserve index helps to identify CMD and allows risk stratification [39, 40].

PET is a well-validated technique that can provide non-invasive, accurate, and reproducible quantification of MBF and CFR in humans, and is thus used for assessment of coronary vasomotor function [41, 42]. Recent PET studies demonstrated that coronary vascular dysfunction, as defined by reduced CFR, is highly prevalent among patients with CAD, [25] increases the severity of inducible myocardial ischemia and subclinical myocardial injury, [43], and identifies patients at high risk for future cardiac events [44]. PET also has the advantage of assessing all three coronary distributions, thus allowing a more accurate assessment of microvascular dysfunction, as CMD has been shown to have a heterogenous distribution over the three vessels [45].

Cardiac magnetic resonance (CMR) has also been used to quantify myocardial perfusion following the injection of a gadolinium-based contrast agent [46]. Advantages of CMR are high spatial resolution, allowing transmural characterization of myocardial blood flow, and the lack of ionizing radiation, along with the ability to perform a comprehensive assessment of cardiovascular structure and function. A decreased response to vasodilator is seen in the subendocardial region in CMD patients and was shown to predict prognosis [47, 48]. A gadolinium-free stress CMR approach using T1 mapping has also been recently proposed for diagnosis of myocardial ischemia with and without obstructive CAD [49].

7.3.2 Invasive Guidewire-Based Techniques for Diagnosis of CMD

Invasive coronary angiography, by combining the ability to exclude obstructive CAD with complementary catheter-based techniques to investigate epicardial and microvascular coronary physiology, is an attractive approach to evaluate patients with CMD [50]. It often involves an interventional procedure where a guidewire-based assessment of coronary blood flow is performed at rest and during interrogation with pharmacological probes, typically adenosine [27, 50]. The procedure is invasive by nature, requires special expertise, and can be time-consuming. However, it has been shown to be safe and effective when performed by experienced interventional operators [51]. Coronary flow reserve (CFR) reflects the ratio of hyperemic flow to basal flow and was first describe by Gould et al. in 1974 [52]. This is also termed the vasodilator capacity and reflects the ability of the coronary circulation to augment blood flow from rest. CFR is calculated using thermodilution as the resting mean transit time divided by hyperemic mean transit time, and an abnormal CFR is defined as ≤ 2 (Fig. 7.2) [25, 53]. Importantly, decreased CFR is associated with increased risk of MACE [15]. CFR reflects the combined vasodilator capacity of the epicardial coronary artery and its subtended microvasculature. Thus, there are some limitations for the use of invasively measured CFR due to its sensitivity to systemic hemodynamics, myocardial contractility, and challenges with establishing true resting coronary blood flow during invasive coronary angiography [54]. Specific

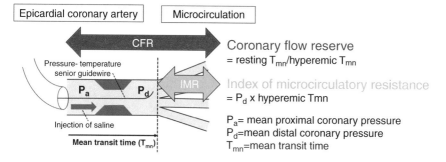

Fig. 7.2 To evaluate relaxation of the coronary artery, a guidewire-based assessment of coronary blood flow is performed at rest and during interrogation with pharmacological probes, typically adenosine. *CFR* coronary flow reserve, *IMR* index of microcirculatory resistance

measures of microvascular resistance are more reproducible and specific and are directly informative about microvascular disease [55]. Index of microvascular resistance (IMR) is calculated as the distal coronary pressure divided by the inverse of the mean transit time during maximal hyperemia [56]. It can be measured by the use of a combined pressure-temperature sensor-tipped coronary guidewire, which allows simultaneous measurement of coronary pressure and hyperemic flow (Fig. 7.2). Increased IMR (e.g. $\geq$25) is representative of CMD and is associated with worse cardiovascular outcomes [57, 58]. Here is the standard measurement technique of IMR [59]. Briefly, systemic administration of heparin (50 ~ 100 IU/kg) and intracoronary nitroglycerin (100 ~ 200 μg) is necessary before measuring IMR. A coronary pressure–temperature sensor guidewire is calibrated, equalized to the guide catheter pressure with the pressure sensor positioned at the tip of the catheter, and advanced to the distal two thirds of the target vessel. For an accurate thermodilution measurement, the sensor needs to be at least 6 cm into the coronary artery. A three-way stopcock and 3-mL syringe are connected to the back of the manifold. The guide catheter is flushed with saline, clearing all contrast, and an operator should pause for a minute to allow coronary flow to return to baseline. If the operator intends to calculate CFR also, then 3 mL of room-temperature saline is briskly injected through the guide catheter under resting conditions, and the console automatically calculates the mean transit time (T_{mn}) at rest. After making the resting measurement, hyperemia is induced by either infusing intravenous adenosine (140 μg·kg^{-1}·min^{-1}) or by injecting intracoronary papaverine (10 ~ 20 mg). During maximal hyperemia, 3 mL of room-temperature saline is briskly injected through the guide catheter, and the hyperemic T_{mn} (T_{mn}Hyp) is measured again as described above. The system allows the operator to examine the T_{mn} curve and calculated time; if the operator is not happy, the value can be replaced with another injection. In some cases, variability in the T_{mn} values can occur, particularly if the guide catheter is moving out of the coronary ostium during saline injection. If all 3 T_{mn} values are <0.25%, then the variability can be ignored because in most cases, IMR will be in the normal range. If T_{mn} is >0.25% and ([the maximum individual T_{mn} value minus the minimum T_{mn} value]/the maximum T_{mn} value×100%) >30%, then the T_{mn} value that is furthest from the mean T_{mn} should be replaced. P_d is measured simultaneously with the same pressure wire during maximal hyperemia, and IMR is calculated as P_d multiplied by T_{mn}Hyp [60].

7.4 Objective Documentation of Coronary Microvascular Spasm

Primary reduction of coronary blood flow caused by spasm of coronary small arteries or arterioles may be the cause of angina at rest. This hypothesis is supported by the careful observations of patients with syndrome X which demonstrated that angina and ischemic ST shift were not always preceded by increments in heart rate [61]. Sinus tachycardia that had caused ischemia during exercise testing did not develop chest pain or ECG change in most instances [61]. The variable threshold for angina symptoms during daily life suggests the presence of circadian variations in vasomotor tone and small vessel hyperconstriction [62]. Mohri et al. prospectively examined a cohort of 117 patients with angina (mostly at rest) and normal or minimally diseased epicardial coronary arteries. In 25% of the patients studied, no epicardial spasm was demonstrated during angina attack on selective coronary arteriography [63]. Chest pain which was similar to patients' previous ones developed in association with ischemic ECG changes and lactate production (an objective marker of myocardial ischemia) spontaneously or following intracoronary acetylcholine. In these patients, the pressure-rate product (an index of myocardial oxygen demand) was comparable between at rest and at the onset of angina. Thus, the decrease in coronary blood flow, rather than increased myocardial oxygen consumption, was a likely explanation for myocardial ischemia. This study suggests that coronary microvascular spasm is the cause of chest pain in a subset of patients with rest angina and normal epicardial coronary arteries. Microvascular constriction and myocardial ischemia as evidenced by ECG change were also provoked by intracoronary infusion of a peptide neurotransmitter, neuropeptide Y [64].

Acetylcholine provocation test should be performed following the guidelines of the Japanese Circulation Society [8]. Briefly, ACh was administered into the coronary artery in a cumulative manner (20, 50, and 100 μg) with careful monitoring of arterial pressure and 12-lead ECG and serial coronary angiograms at 1-min intervals. Calcium channel blockers, long-acting nitrates, and nicorandil need to be discontinued at least 48 h before the provocation test. To determine whether multivessel coronary spasm would develop, the authors first perform ACh provocation test for the LCA in a cumulative manner (20, 50, and 100 mg). If the test for the LCA is negative or ACh-induced spasms in the LCA resolves spontaneously, ACh is then injected into the right coronary artery in a cumulative manner (20 and 50 mg). When coronary spasm is induced, 5 mg of isosorbide dinitrate (ISDN) is injected into the responsible coronary artery. Additionally, to evaluate the presence of coronary microvascular spasm, lactate production during myocardial ischemia induced by ACh provocation test is recommended. Myocardial lactate extraction ratio is calculated as the ratio of the coronary arterial–venous difference in lactate concentration to the arterial concentration. Myocardial lactate production defined by negative myocardial lactate extraction ratio is considered to be highly sensitive to myocardial ischemia [65]. Microvascular spasm (MVS) is defined as myocardial lactate production despite the absence of angiographically demonstrable epicardial spasm throughout ACh provocation test or prior to the occurrence of epicardial coronary spasm following intracoronary injections of ACh [66]. At 1 min after each dose of ACh is given to LCA, paired samples of 1 mL of blood are collected from the left coronary ostium and the coronary sinus for measurement of lactate concentrations, which are immediately determined with a calibrated automatic lactate analyzer. We usually evaluate lactate production during ACh provocation test only in the LCA, as the great coronary sinus drains blood from the LCAs but not from the right coronary artery.

7.5 Biomarkers of Coronary Microvascular Dysfunction

The causes of CMD appear to be heterogeneous [14, 17]. Classical coronary risk factors are associated with impaired coronary microvascular dilatation and enhanced coronary microvascular constriction [67]. Recently, low-grade inflammation attracts much attention in the pathogenesis of CMD, as CRP levels correlate with the frequency of angina attacks and impairment of coronary microvascular dilatation in patients with syndrome X [68]. Although the importance of CMD has been emerging, reliable biomarkers for CMD still remain to be developed. Serotonin is released from aggregating platelets, causing vasoconstriction and platelet aggregation with cyclic flow reduction [69]. Several clinical studies previously addressed the relationship between systemic serotonin concentrations and coronary vasomotor dysfunction in a small number of patients with inconsistent results [70, 71]. We examined the potential usefulness of plasma concentration of serotonin to diagnose CMD [72]. CMD was defined as myocardial lactate production without or prior to the occurrence of epicardial coronary spasm during acetylcholine provocation test. Although no statistical difference in plasma concentration of serotonin [median (inter-quartile range) nmol/L] was noted between the vasospastic angina (VSA) and non-VSA groups, it was significantly higher in patients with MVS compared with those without it (Fig. 7.3). Among the four groups classified according to the

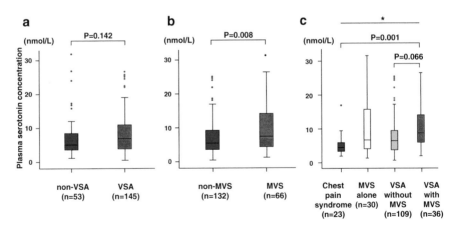

Fig. 7.3 (**a**) Plasma concentrations of serotonin were compatible between the VSA and the non-VSA groups. Results are expressed as box-and-whisker plots; the central box covers the interquartile range, with the median indicated by the line within the box. The whiskers extend to the most extreme values within 1.5 interquartile ranges. More extreme values are plotted individually. (**b**) Plasma concentrations of serotonin were higher in patients with MVS than in those without it. (**c**) Plasma serotonin concentrations of the four groups classified according to the presence or absence of VSA and MVS are shown. The serotonin concentrations were significantly higher in the VSA with MVS group than in the chest pain syndrome group by Steel-Dwass test. $*P < 0.01$ for the difference in plasma concentrations of serotonin among the four groups by Kruskal-Wallis test. *VSA* vasospastic angina, *MVS* coronary microvascular spasm. (Reproduced from Odaka et al. [72])

presence or absence of VSA and MVS, serotonin concentration was highest in the VSA with MVS group (Fig. 7.3). Importantly, there was a positive correlation between plasma serotonin concentration and baseline TIMI frame count, a marker of coronary vascular resistance [73]. The classification and regression trees analysis showed that plasma serotonin concentration of 9.55 nmol/L was the first discriminator to stratify the risk for the presence of MVS. In multivariable analysis, serotonin concentration greater than the cut-off value had the largest odds ratio in the prediction of MVS [73]. These results suggest that plasma concentration of serotonin may be a novel biomarker to dissect MVS from epicardial coronary artery spasm.

7.6   Comprehensive Evaluation of the Coronary Functional Abnormalities

Although the importance of coronary functional abnormalities (epicardial coronary spasm and CMD) in patients with chest pain and non-obstructive CAD has been emerging, their pathogenesis and prognostic implications remain to be fully elucidated. Lee et al. showed that integration of microvascular assessment by both CFR and IMR can improve the accuracy of prognostic prediction for patients with high FFR; however, no attention was paid to epicardial coronary spasm [58]. Recent studies demonstrated that VSA is frequently noted in Caucasian patients with chest pain and non-obstructive CAD and those with acute myocardial infarction and non-obstructive CAD than ever thought [74, 75]. Thus, attention should always be paid to possible involvement of epicardial coronary spasm in patients with chest pain and non-obstructive CAD. Thus, we examined the significance of coronary functional abnormalities in a comprehensive manner for both epicardial and microvascular coronary arteries in patients with angina and non-obstructive CAD [76]. Recently, the combined invasive assessment of coronary vasoconstrictor as well as vasodilator abnormalities has been titled interventional diagnostic procedure (IDP) [50, 77]. When examining patients with chest pain and non-obstructive CAD, we routinely performed intracoronary ACh testing for detection of coronary spasm as well as coronary flow reserve and microvascular resistance assessment in response to adenosine using a coronary pressure–temperature sensor guidewire. Then, we prospectively enrolled consecutive patients, who underwent ACh provocation test for coronary spasm and measurement of IMR to evaluate coronary microvascular function, and followed them. Multivariable analysis revealed that IMR correlated with the incidence of cardiac events and receiver-operating characteristics curve analysis identified IMR of 18.0 as the optimal cut-off value. Importantly, there were substantial overlaps of coronary functional abnormality in various combinations among VSA, low CFR (CFR < 2.0), and high IMR (IMR $\geq$ 18) (Fig. 7.4). Among the four groups based on the cut-off value of IMR and the presence of VSA, the Kaplan-Meier survival analysis showed a significantly worse prognosis in the group with high IMR ($\geq$18.0) and VSA compared with other groups (Fig. 7.5). Importantly, intracoronary administration of fasudil, a Rho-kinase inhibitor, significantly

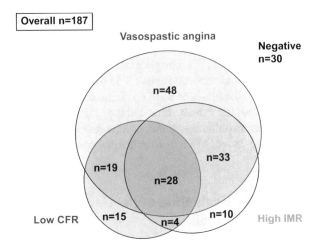

Fig. 7.4 Among 187 patients, 128 (68.4%) were diagnosed as having VSA by ACh provocation test. Furthermore, 66 (35.3%) had low CFR (CFR < 2.0) and 75 (40.1%) high IMR (IMR ≥ 18). Thus, more than half of VSA patients had microvascular functional abnormalities, including low CFR (n = 19, 10.2%), high IMR (n = 33, 17.6%), and both of them (n = 28, 15.0%). *CFR* coronary flow reserve, *IMR* index of microcirculatory resistance, *VSA* vasospastic angina. (Reproduced from Suda et al. [76])

ameliorated IMR in the VSA patients with increased IMR. These results indicate that in patients with angina and non-obstructive CAD, coexistence of epicardial coronary spasm and increased microvascular resistance is associated with worse prognosis, for which Rho-kinase activation may be involved. Thus, comprehensive assessment of coronary functional abnormalities, including epicardial coronary spasm and increased microvascular resistance, could be useful for risk stratification of patients with angina and non-obstructive CAD. Furthermore, Rho-kinase inhibition with fasudil may be useful for the treatment of those coronary functional abnormalities.

There is a critical missing link between the use of relevant diagnostic tests of coronary artery function and therapeutic agents with proven efficiency and health outcomes of patients with angina without obstructive CAD. This gap in evidence was recently addressed in CORonary MICrovascular Angina randomized controlled trial (CorMicA), which tested whether an IDP linked to stratified medicine improves health status in patients with ischemia but non-obstructive CAD [77]. CorMicA trial demonstrated that vasoreactivity testing with ACh and measurement of CFR and IMR can be used to guide medication therapy in patients without non-obstructive CAD. Moreover, the stratified medical therapy leads to marked and sustained angina improvement and better quality of life at 1 year following invasive coronary angiography [78]. Based on these results of CorMicA, it was suggested that the IDP could provide the most comprehensive coronary vasomotor assessment.

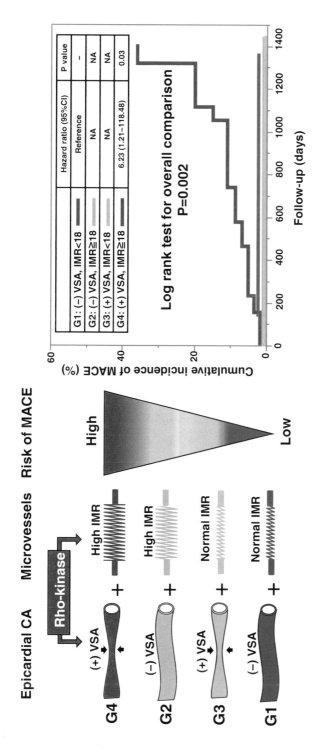

Fig. 7.5 In patients with chest pain and unobstructive CAD, coexistence of VSA (epicardial coronary spasm) and high IMR (microvascular resistance) is associated with worse prognosis, for which Rho-kinase activation may be involved. *CA* coronary artery, *IMR* index of microcirculatory resistance, *VSA* vasospastic angina. (Reproduced from Suda et al. [76])

References

1. Patel MR, Peterson ED, Dai D, Brennan JM, Redberg RF, Anderson HV, Brindis RG, Douglas PS. Low diagnostic yield of elective coronary angiography. N Engl J Med. 2010;362(10):886–95. https://doi.org/10.1056/NEJMoa0907272.
2. Pepine CJ, Ferdinand KC, Shaw LJ, Light-McGroary KA, Shah RU, Gulati M, Duvernoy C, Walsh MN, Bairey Merz CN, ACC CVD in Women Committee. Emergence of non-obstructive coronary artery disease: a woman's problem and need for change in definition on angiography. J Am Coll Cardiol. 2015;66(17):1918–33. https://doi.org/10.1016/j.jacc.2015.08.876.
3. Shaw LJ, Bairey Merz CN, Pepine CJ, Reis SE, Bittner V, Kelsey SF, Olson M, Johnson BD, Mankad S, Sharaf BL, Rogers WJ, Wessel TR, Arant CB, Pohost GM, Lerman A, Quyyumi AA, Sopko G, WISE Investigators. Insights from the NHLBI-sponsored Women's ischemia syndrome evaluation (WISE) study: part I: gender differences in traditional and novel risk factors, symptom evaluation, and gender-optimized diagnostic strategies. J Am Coll Cardiol. 2006;47(3 Suppl):S4–S20. https://doi.org/10.1016/j.jacc.2005.01.072.
4. Shimokawa H. 2014 Williams Harvey lecture: importance of coronary vasomotion abnormalities-from bench to bedside. Eur Heart J. 2014;35(45):3180–93. https://doi.org/10.1093/eurheartj/ehu427.
5. Takagi Y, Yasuda S, Tsunoda R, Ogata Y, Seki A, Sumiyoshi T, Matsui M, Goto T, Tanabe Y, Sueda S, Sato T, Ogawa S, Kubo N, Momomura S, Ogawa H, Shimokawa H, Japanese Coronary Spasm Association. Clinical characteristics and long-term prognosis of vasospastic angina patients who survived out-of-hospital cardiac arrest: multicenter registry study of the Japanese Coronary Spasm Association. Circ Arrhythm Electrophysiol. 2011;4(3):295–302. https://doi.org/10.1161/CIRCEP.110.959809.
6. Takagi Y, Takahashi J, Yasuda S, Miyata S, Tsunoda R, Ogata Y, Seki A, Sumiyoshi T, Matsui M, Goto T, Tanabe Y, Sueda S, Sato T, Ogawa S, Kubo N, Momomura S, Ogawa H, Shimokawa H, Japanese Coronary Spasm Association. Prognostic stratification of patients with vasospastic angina: a comprehensive clinical risk score developed by the Japanese Coronary Spasm Association. J Am Coll Cardiol. 2013;62(13):1144–53. https://doi.org/10.1016/j.jacc.2013.07.018.
7. Takahashi J, Nihei T, Takagi Y, Miyata S, Odaka Y, Tsunoda R, Seki A, Sumiyoshi T, Matsui M, Goto T, Tanabe Y, Sueda S, Momomura S, Yasuda S, Ogawa H, Shimokawa H, Japanese Coronary Spasm Association. Prognostic impact of chronic nitrate therapy in patients with vasospastic angina: multicentre registry study of the Japanese coronary spasm association. Eur Heart J. 2015;36(4):228–37. https://doi.org/10.1093/eurheartj/ehu313.
8. JCS Joint Working Group. Guidelines for diagnosis and treatment of patients with vasospastic angina (Coronary Spastic Angina) (JCS 2013). Circ J. 2014;78(11):2779–801. https://doi.org/10.1253/circj.cj-66-0098.
9. Beltrame JF, Crea F, Kaski JC, Ogawa H, Ong P, Sechtem U, Shimokawa H, Bairey Merz CN, Coronary Vasomotion Disorders International Study Group (COVADIS). International standardization of diagnostic criteria for vasospastic angina. Eur Heart J. 2017;38(33):2565–8. https://doi.org/10.1093/eurheartj/ehv351.
10. Sueda S, Kohno H, Ochi T, Uraoka T, Tsunemitsu K. Overview of the pharmacological spasm provocation test: comparisons between acetylcholine and ergonovine. J Cardiol. 2017;69(1):57–65. https://doi.org/10.1016/j.jjcc.2016.09.012.
11. Zaya M, Mehta PK, Merz CN. Provocative testing for coronary reactivity and spasm. J Am Coll Cardiol. 2014;63(2):103–9. https://doi.org/10.1016/j.jacc.2013.10.038.
12. Kikuchi Y, Yasuda S, Aizawa K, Tsuburaya R, Ito Y, Takeda M, Nakayama M, Ito K, Takahashi J, Shimokawa H. Enhanced Rho-kinase activity in circulating neutrophils of patients with vasospastic angina: a possible biomarker for diagnosis and disease activity assessment. J Am Coll Cardiol. 2011;58(12):1231–7. https://doi.org/10.1016/j.jacc.2011.05.046.

13. Nihei T, Takahashi J, Tsuburaya R, Ito Y, Shiroto T, Hao K, Takagi Y, Matsumoto Y, Nakayama M, Miyata S, Sakata Y, Ito K, Shimokawa H. Circadian variation of Rho-kinase activity in circulating leukocytes of patients with vasospastic angina. Circ J. 2014;78(5):1183–90. https://doi.org/10.1253/circj.cj-13-1458.
14. Crea F, Camici PG, Bairey Merz CN. Coronary microvascular dysfunction: an update. Eur Heart J. 2014;35(17):1101–11. https://doi.org/10.1093/eurheartj/eht513.
15. Pepine CJ, Anderson RD, Sharaf BL, Reis SE, Smith KM, Handberg EM, Johnson BD, Sopko G, Bairey Merz CN. Coronary microvascular reactivity to adenosine predicts adverse outcome in women evaluated for suspected ischemia results from the National Heart, Lung and Blood Institute WISE (Women's ischemia syndrome evaluation) study. J Am Coll Cardiol. 2010;55(25):2825–32. https://doi.org/10.1016/j.jacc.2010.01.054.
16. Taqueti VR, Di Carli MF. Coronary microvascular disease pathogenic mechanisms and therapeutic options: JACC state-of-the-art review. J Am Coll Cardiol. 2018;72(21):2625–41. https://doi.org/10.1016/j.jacc.2018.09.042.
17. Camici PG, d'Amati G, Rimoldi O. Coronary microvascular dysfunction: mechanisms and functional assessment. Nat Rev Cardiol. 2015;12(1):48–62. https://doi.org/10.1038/nrcardio.2014.160.
18. Lamendola P, Lanza GA, Spinelli A, Sgueglia GA, Di Monaco A, Barone L, Sestito A, Crea F. Long-term prognosis of patients with cardiac syndrome X. Int J Cardiol. 2010;140(2):197–9. https://doi.org/10.1016/j.ijcard.2008.11.026.
19. Lanza GA, Crea F. Primary coronary microvascular dysfunction: clinical presentation, pathophysiology, and management. Circulation. 2010;121(21):2317–25. https://doi.org/10.1161/CIRCULATIONAHA.109.900191.
20. Kanatsuka H, Eastham CL, Marcus ML, Lamping KG. Effects of nitroglycerin on the coronary microcirculation in normal and ischemic myocardium. J Cardiovasc Pharmacol. 1992;19(5):755–63.
21. Gulati M, Shaw LJ, Bairey Merz CN. Myocardial ischemia in women: lessons from the NHLBI WISE study. Clin Cardiol. 2012;35(3):141–8. https://doi.org/10.1002/clc.21966.
22. Mygind ND, Michelsen MM, Pena A, Frestad D, Dose N, Aziz A, Faber R, Høst N, Gustafsson I, Hansen PR, Hansen HS, Bairey Merz CN, Kastrup J, Prescott E. Coronary microvascular function and cardiovascular risk factors in women with angina pectoris and no obstructive coronary artery disease: the iPOWER study. J Am Heart Assoc. 2016;5(3):e003064. https://doi.org/10.1161/JAHA.115.003064.
23. Pijls NH, De Bruyne B, Bech GJ, Liistro F, Heyndrickx GR, Bonnier HJ, Koolen JJ. Coronary pressure measurement to assess the hemodynamic significance of serial stenoses within one coronary artery: validation in humans. Circulation. 2000;102(19):2371–7. https://doi.org/10.1161/01.cir.102.19.2371.
24. Ong P, Camici PG, Beltrame JF, Crea F, Shimokawa H, Sechtem U, Kaski JC, Noel Bairey Merz C, Coronary Vasomotion Disorders International Study Group (COVADIS). International standardization of diagnostic criteria for microvascular angina. Int J Cardiol. 2018;250:16–20. https://doi.org/10.1016/j.ijcard.2017.08.068.
25. Murthy VL, Naya M, Taqueti VR, Foster CR, Gaber M, Hainer J, Dorbala S, Blankstein R, Rimoldi O, Camici PG, Di Carli MF. Effects of sex on coronary microvascular dysfunction and cardiac outcomes. Circulation. 2014;129(24):2518–27. https://doi.org/10.1161/CIRCULATIONAHA.113.008507.
26. Bairey Merz CN, Handberg EM, Shufelt CL, Mehta PK, Minissian MB, Wei J, Thomson LE, Berman DS, Shaw LJ, Petersen JW, Brown GH, Anderson RD, Shuster JJ, Cook-Wiens G, Rogatko A, Pepine CJ. A randomized, placebo-controlled trial of late Na current inhibition (ranolazine) in coronary microvascular dysfunction (CMD): impact on angina and myocardial perfusion reserve. Eur Heart J. 2016;37(19):1504–13. https://doi.org/10.1093/eurheartj/ehv647.
27. Sara JD, Widmer RJ, Matsuzawa Y, Lennon RJ, Lerman LO, Lerman A. Prevalence of coronary microvascular dysfunction among patients with chest pain and nonobstructive coronary

artery disease. JACC Cardiovasc Interv. 2015;8(11):1445–53. https://doi.org/10.1016/j.jcin.2015.06.017.

28. Shah NR, Cheezum MK, Veeranna V, Horgan SJ, Taqueti VR, Murthy VL, Foster C, Hainer J, Daniels KM, Rivero J, Shah AM, Stone PH, Morrow DA, Steigner ML, Dorbala S, Blankstein R, Di Carli MF. Ranolazine in symptomatic diabetic patients without obstructive coronary artery disease: impact on microvascular and diastolic function. J Am Heart Assoc. 2017;6(5):e005027. https://doi.org/10.1161/JAHA.116.005027.

29. Taqueti VR, Solomon SD, Shah AM, Desai AS, Groarke JD, Osborne MT, Hainer J, Bibbo CF, Dorbala S, Blankstein R, Di Carli MF. Coronary microvascular dysfunction and future risk of heart failure with preserved ejection fraction. Eur Heart J. 2018;39(10):840–9. https://doi.org/10.1093/eurheartj/ehx721.

30. Webb CM, Collins P, Di Mario C. Normal coronary physiology assessed by intracoronary Doppler ultrasound. Herz. 2005;30(1):8–16. https://doi.org/10.1007/s00059-005-2647-z.

31. Layland J, Carrick D, Lee M, Oldroyd K, Berry C. Adenosine: physiology, pharmacology, and clinical applications. JACC Cardiovasc Interv. 2014;7(6):581–91. https://doi.org/10.1016/j.jcin.2014.02.009.

32. McGuinness ME, Talbert RL. Pharmacologic stress testing: experience with dipyridamole, adenosine, and dobutamine. Am J Hosp Pharm. 1994;51(3):328–46; quiz 404-5

33. Loffler AI, Bourque JM. Coronary microvascular dysfunction, microvascular angina, and management. Curr Cardiol Rep. 2016;18(1):1. https://doi.org/10.1007/s11886-015-0682-9.

34. Saraste M, Koskenvuo J, Knuuti J, Toikka J, Laine H, Niemi P, Sakuma H, Hartiala J. Coronary flow reserve: measurement with transthoracic Doppler echocardiography is reproducible and comparable with positron emission tomography. Clin Physiol. 2001;21(1):114–22. https://doi.org/10.1046/j.1365-2281.2001.00296.x.

35. Caiati C, Montaldo C, Zedda N, Montisci R, Ruscazio M, Lai G, Cadeddu M, Meloni L, Iliceto S. Validation of a new noninvasive method (contrast-enhanced transthoracic second harmonic echo Doppler) for the evaluation of coronary flow reserve: comparison with intracoronary Doppler flow wire. J Am Coll Cardiol. 1999;34(4):1193–200. https://doi.org/10.1016/s0735-1097(99)00342-3.

36. Rigo F, Richieri M, Pasanisi E, Cutaia V, Zanella C, Della Valentina P, Di Pede F, Raviele A, Picano E. Usefulness of coronary flow reserve over regional wall motion when added to dual-imaging dipyridamole echocardiography. Am J Cardiol. 2003;91(3):269–73. https://doi.org/10.1016/s0002-9149(02)03153-3.

37. Kaul S. Myocardial contrast echocardiography: a 25-year retrospective. Circulation. 2008;118(3):291–308. https://doi.org/10.1161/CIRCULATIONAHA.107.747303.

38. Vogel R, Indermuhle A, Reinhardt J, Meier P, Siegrist PT, Namdar M, Kaufmann PA, Seiler C. The quantification of absolute myocardial perfusion in humans by contrast echocardiography: algorithm and validation. J Am Coll Cardiol. 2005;45(5):754–62. https://doi.org/10.1016/j.jacc.2004.11.044.

39. Gan LM, Svedlund S, Wittfeldt A, Eklund C, Gao S, Matejka G, Jeppsson A, Albertsson P, Omerovic E, Lerman A. Incremental value of transthoracic Doppler echocardiography-assessed coronary flow reserve in patients with suspected myocardial ischemia undergoing myocardial perfusion scintigraphy. J Am Heart Assoc. 2017;6(4):e004875. https://doi.org/10.1161/JAHA.116.004875.

40. Gurudevan SV, Nelson MD, Rader F, Tang X, Lewis J, Johannes J, Belcik JT, Elashoff RM, Lindner JR, Victor RG. Cocaine-induced vasoconstriction in the human coronary microcirculation: new evidence from myocardial contrast echocardiography. Circulation. 2013;128(6):598–604. https://doi.org/10.1161/CIRCULATIONAHA.113.002937.

41. Camici PG, Rimoldi OE. The clinical value of myocardial blood flow measurement. J Nucl Med. 2009;50(7):1076–87. https://doi.org/10.2967/jnumed.108.054478.

42. Gould KL, Johnson NP, Bateman TM, Beanlands RS, Bengel FM, Bober R, Camici PG, Cerqueira MD, BJW C, Di Carli MF, Dorbala S, Gewirtz H, Gropler RJ, Kaufmann PA, Knaapen P, Knuuti J, Merhige ME, Rentrop KP, Ruddy TD, Schelbert HR, Schindler TH, Schwaiger M,

Sdringola S, Vitarello J, Williams KA Sr, Gordon D, Dilsizian V, Narula J. Anatomic versus physiologic assessment of coronary artery disease. Role of coronary flow reserve, fractional flow reserve, and positron emission tomography imaging in revascularization decision-making. J Am Coll Cardiol. 2013;62(18):1639–53. https://doi.org/10.1016/j.jacc.2013.07.076.

43. Taqueti VR, Everett BM, Murthy VL, Gaber M, Foster CR, Hainer J, Blankstein R, Dorbala S, Di Carli MF. Interaction of impaired coronary flow reserve and cardiomyocyte injury on adverse cardiovascular outcomes in patients without overt coronary artery disease. Circulation. 2015;131(6):528–35. https://doi.org/10.1161/CIRCULATIONAHA.114.009716.

44. Gupta A, Taqueti VR, van de Hoef TP, Bajaj NS, Bravo PE, Murthy VL, Osborne MT, Seidelmann SB, Vita T, Bibbo CF, Harrington M, Hainer J, Rimoldi O, Dorbala S, Bhatt DL, Blankstein R, Camici PG, Di Carli MF. Integrated noninvasive physiological assessment of coronary circulatory function and impact on cardiovascular mortality in patients with stable coronary artery disease. Circulation. 2017;136(24):2325–36. https://doi.org/10.1161/CIRCULATIONAHA.117.029992.

45. Marroquin OC, Holubkov R, Edmundowicz D, Rickens C, Pohost G, Buchthal S, Pepine CJ, Sopko G, Sembrat RC, Meltzer CC, Reis SE. Heterogeneity of microvascular dysfunction in women with chest pain not attributable to coronary artery disease: implications for clinical practice. Am Heart J. 2003;145(4):628–35. https://doi.org/10.1067/mhj.2003.95.

46. Feher A, Sinusas AJ. Quantitative assessment of coronary microvascular function: dynamic single-photon emission computed tomography, positron emission tomography, ultrasound, computed tomography, and magnetic resonance imaging. Circ Cardiovasc Imaging. 2017;10(8):e006427. https://doi.org/10.1161/CIRCIMAGING.117.006427.

47. Panting JR, Gatehouse PD, Yang GZ, Grothues F, Firmin DN, Collins P, Pennell DJ. Abnormal subendocardial perfusion in cardiac syndrome X detected by cardiovascular magnetic resonance imaging. N Engl J Med. 2002;346(25):1948–53. https://doi.org/10.1056/NEJMoa012369.

48. Doyle M, Weinberg N, Pohost GM, Bairey Merz CN, Shaw LJ, Sopko G, Fuisz A, Rogers WJ, Walsh EG, Johnson BD, Sharaf BL, Pepine CJ, Mankad S, Reis SE, Vido DA, Rayarao G, Bittner V, Tauxe L, Olson MB, Kelsey SF, Biederman RW. Prognostic value of global MR myocardial perfusion imaging in women with suspected myocardial ischemia and no obstructive coronary disease: results from the NHLBI-sponsored WISE (Women's Ischemia Syndrome Evaluation) study. JACC Cardiovasc Imaging. 2010;3(10):1030–6. https://doi.org/10.1016/j.jcmg.2010.07.008.

49. Liu A, Wijesurendra RS, Liu JM, Forfar JC, Channon KM, Jerosch-Herold M, Jerosch-Herold M, Piechnik SK, Neubauer S, Kharbanda RK, Ferreira VM. Diagnosis of microvascular angina using cardiac magnetic resonance. J Am Coll Cardiol. 2018;71(9):969–79. https://doi.org/10.1016/j.jacc.2017.12.046.

50. Ford TJ, Berry C. How to diagnose and manage angina without obstructive coronary artery disease: lessons from the British Heart Foundation CorMicA Trial. Interv Cardiol. 2019;14(2):76–82. https://doi.org/10.15420/icr.2019.04.R1.

51. Wei J, Mehta PK, Johnson BD, Samuels B, Kar S, Anderson RD, Azarbal B, Petersen J, Sharaf B, Handberg E, Shufelt C, Kothawade K, Sopko G, Lerman A, Shaw L, Kelsey SF, Pepine CJ, Merz CN. Safety of coronary reactivity testing in women with no obstructive coronary artery disease: results from the NHLBI-sponsored WISE (Women's ischemia syndrome evaluation) study. JACC Cardiovasc Interv. 2012;5(6):646–53. https://doi.org/10.1016/j.jcin.2012.01.023.

52. Gould KL, Lipscomb K, Hamilton GW. Physiologic basis for assessing critical coronary stenosis. Instantaneous flow response and regional distribution during coronary hyperemia as measures of coronary flow reserve. Am J Cardiol. 1974;33(1):87–94. https://doi.org/10.1016/0002-9149(74)90743-7.

53. Pijls NH, De Bruyne B, Smith L, Aarnoudse W, Barbato E, Bartunek J, Bech GJ, Van De Vosse F. Coronary thermodilution to assess flow reserve: validation in humans. Circulation. 2002;105(21):2482–6. https://doi.org/10.1161/01.cir.0000017199.09457.3d.

54. McGinn AL, White CW, Wilson RF. Interstudy variability of coronary flow reserve. Influence of heart rate, arterial pressure, and ventricular preload. Circulation. 1990;81(4):1319–30. https://doi.org/10.1161/01.cir.81.4.1319.

55. Ford TJ, Corcoran D, Berry C. Coronary artery disease: physiology and prognosis. Eur Heart J. 2017;38(25):1990–2. https://doi.org/10.1093/eurheartj/ehx226.

56. Fearon WF, Balsam LB, Farouque HM, Caffarelli AD, Robbins RC, Fitzgerald PJ, Yock PG, Yeung AC. Novel index for invasively assessing the coronary microcirculation. Circulation. 2003;107(25):3129–32. https://doi.org/10.1161/01.CIR.0000080700.98607.D1.

57. Lee BK, Lim HS, Fearon WF, Yong AS, Yamada R, Tanaka S, Lee DP, Yeung AC, Tremmel JA. Invasive evaluation of patients with angina in the absence of obstructive coronary artery disease. Circulation. 2015;131(12):1054–60. https://doi.org/10.1161/CIRCULATIONAHA.114.012636.

58. Lee JM, Jung JH, Hwang D, Park J, Fan Y, Na SH, Doh JH, Nam CW, Shin ES, Koo BK. Coronary flow reserve and microcirculatory resistance in patients with intermediate coronary stenosis. J Am Coll Cardiol. 2016;67(10):1158–69. https://doi.org/10.1016/j.jacc.2015.12.053.

59. Fearon WF, Kobayashi Y. Invasive assessment of the coronary microvasculature: the index of microcirculatory resistance. Circ Cardiovasc Interv. 2017;10(12):e005361. https://doi.org/10.1161/CIRCINTERVENTIONS.117.005361.

60. Ng MK, Yeung AC, Fearon WF. Invasive assessment of the coronary microcirculation: superior reproducibility and less hemodynamic dependence of index of microcirculatory resistance compared with coronary flow reserve. Circulation. 2006;113(17):2054–61. https://doi.org/10.1161/CIRCULATIONAHA.105.603522.

61. Kaski JC, Crea F, Nihoyannopoulos P, Hackett D, Maseri A. Transient myocardial ischemia during daily life in patients with syndrome X. Am J Cardiol. 1986;58(13):1242–7. https://doi.org/10.1016/0002-9149(86)90390-5.

62. Lanza GA, Manzoli A, Pasceri V, Colonna G, Cianflone D, Crea F, Maseri A. Ischemic-like ST-segment changes during Holter monitoring in patients with angina pectoris and normal coronary arteries but negative exercise testing. Am J Cardiol. 1997;79(1):1–6. https://doi.org/10.1016/s0002-9149(96)00666-2.

63. Mohri M, Koyanagi M, Egashira K, Tagawa H, Ichiki T, Shimokawa H, Takeshita A. Angina pectoris caused by coronary microvascular spasm. Lancet. 1998;351(9110):1165–9. https://doi.org/10.1016/S0140-6736(97)07329-7.

64. Clarke JG, Davies GJ, Kerwin R, Hackett D, Larkin S, Dawbarn D, Lee Y, Bloom SR, Yacoub M, Maseri A. Coronary artery infusion of neuropeptide Y in patients with angina pectoris. Lancet. 1987;1(8541):1057–9. https://doi.org/10.1016/s0140-6736(87)90483-1.

65. Sun H, Mohri M, Shimokawa H, Usui M, Urakami L, Takeshita A. Coronary microvascular spasm causes myocardial ischemia in patients with vasospastic angina. J Am Coll Cardiol. 2002;39(5):847–51. https://doi.org/10.1016/s0735-1097(02)01690-x.

66. Mohri M, Shimokawa H, Hirakawa Y, Masumoto A, Takeshita A. Rho-kinase inhibition with intracoronary fasudil prevents myocardial ischemia in patients with coronary microvascular spasm. J Am Coll Cardiol. 2003;41(1):15–9. https://doi.org/10.1016/s0735-1097(02)02632-3.

67. Chen C, Wei J, AlBadri A, Zarrini P, Bairey Merz CN. Coronary microvascular dysfunction- epidemiology, pathogenesis, prognosis, diagnosis, risk factors and therapy. Circ J. 2016;81(1):3–11. https://doi.org/10.1253/circj.CJ-16-1002.

68. Cosin-Sales J, Pizzi C, Brown S, Kaski JC. C-reactive protein, clinical presentation, and ischemic activity in patients with chest pain and normal coronary angiograms. J Am Coll Cardiol. 2003;41(9):1468–74. https://doi.org/10.1016/s0735-1097(03)00243-2.

69. Golino P, Ashton JH, Buja LM, Rosolowsky M, Taylor AL, McNatt J, Campbell WB, Willerson JT. Local platelet activation causes vasoconstriction of large epicardial canine coronary arteries in vivo. Thromboxane A2 and serotonin are possible mediators. Circulation. 1989;79(1):154–66. https://doi.org/10.1161/01.cir.79.1.154.

70. Figueras J, Domingo E, Cortadellas J, Padilla F, Dorado DG, Segura R, Galard R, Soler JS. Comparison of plasma serotonin levels in patients with variant angina pectoris versus healed myocardial infarction. Am J Cardiol. 2005;96(2):204–7. https://doi.org/10.1016/j.amjcard.2005.03.044.

71. Murakami Y, Ishinaga Y, Sano K, Murakami R, Kinoshita Y, Kitamura J, Kobayashi K, Okada S, Matsubara K, Shimada T, Morioka S. Increased serotonin release across the coronary bed during a nonischemic interval in patients with vasospastic angina. Clin Cardiol. 1996;19(6):473–6. https://doi.org/10.1002/clc.4960190606.

72. Odaka Y, Takahashi J, Tsuburaya R, Nishimiya K, Hao K, Matsumoto Y, Ito K, Sakata Y, Miyata S, Manita D, Hirowatari Y, Shimokawa H. Plasma concentration of serotonin is a novel biomarker for coronary microvascular dysfunction in patients with suspected angina and unobstructive coronary arteries. Eur Heart J. 2017;38(7):489–96. https://doi.org/10.1093/eurheartj/ehw448.

73. Sun H, Fukumoto Y, Ito A, Shimokawa H, Sunagawa K. Coronary microvascular dysfunction in patients with microvascular angina: analysis by TIMI frame count. J Cardiovasc Pharmacol. 2005;46(5):622–6. https://doi.org/10.1097/01.fjc.0000181291.96086.ae.

74. Ong P, Athanasiadis A, Borgulya G, Mahrholdt H, Kaski JC, Sechtem U. High prevalence of a pathological response to acetylcholine testing in patients with stable angina pectoris and unobstructed coronary arteries. The ACOVA study (abnormal COronary VAsomotion in patients with stable angina and unobstructed coronary arteries). J Am Coll Cardiol. 2012;59(7):655–62. https://doi.org/10.1016/j.jacc.2011.11.015.

75. Montone RA, Niccoli G, Fracassi F, Russo M, Gurgoglione F, Camma G, Lanza GA, Crea F. Patients with acute myocardial infarction and non-obstructive coronary arteries: safety and prognostic relevance of invasive coronary provocative tests. Eur Heart J. 2018;39(2):91–8. https://doi.org/10.1093/eurheartj/ehx667.

76. Suda A, Takahashi J, Hao K, Kikuchi Y, Shindo T, Ikeda S, Sato K, Sugisawa J, Matsumoto Y, Miyata S, Sakata Y, Shimokawa H. Coronary functional abnormalities in patients with angina and nonobstructive coronary artery disease. J Am Coll Cardiol. 2019;74(19):2350–60. https://doi.org/10.1016/j.jacc.2019.08.1056.

77. Ford TJ, Stanley B, Good R, Rocchiccioli P, McEntegart M, Watkins S, Eteiba H, Shaukat A, Lindsay M, Robertson K, Hood S, McGeoch R, McDade R, Yii E, Sidik N, McCartney P, Corcoran D, Collison D, Rush C, McConnachie A, Touyz RM, Oldroyd KG, Berry C. Stratified medical therapy using invasive coronary function testing in angina: The CorMicA Trial. J Am Coll Cardiol. 2018;72(23 Pt A):2841–55. https://doi.org/10.1016/j.jacc.2018.09.006.

78. Ford TJ, Stanley B, Sidik N, Good R, Rocchiccioli P, McEntegart M, Watkins S, Eteiba H, Shaukat A, Lindsay M, Robertson K, Hood S, McGeoch R, McDade R, Yii E, McCartney P, Corcoran D, Collison D, Rush C, Sattar N, McConnachie A, Touyz RM, Oldroyd KG, Berry C. 1-year outcomes of angina management guided by invasive coronary function testing (CorMicA). JACC Cardiovasc Interv. 2020;13(1):33–45. https://doi.org/10.1016/j.jcin.2019.11.001.

Chapter 8
Treatment of Coronary Microvascular Dysfunction

Jun Takahashi and Hiroaki Shimokawa

Abstract Patients with ischemia and non-obstructive coronary artery (INOCA) often have coronary microvascular dysfunction (CMD), and they are at high risk for adverse cardiac events. Nevertheless, the management of CMD represents a major unmet need because the lack of large, randomized studies makes it difficult to generate evidence-based recommendations. Recently, it was demonstrated that stratified medical therapy guided by an interventional diagnostic procedure improves health status of patients with INOCA. Accordingly, the latest guidelines state that treatment of CMD should address the dominant mechanism of microcirculatory dysfunction. In patients with impaired microcirculatory conductance and a negative acetylcholine (ACh) provocation test, beta-blockers, ACE inhibitors, and statins, along with lifestyle modifications and weight loss, are indicated. On the other hand, patients developing ECG changes and angina in response to ACh testing but without severe epicardial coronary vasoconstriction (all suggestive of microvascular spasm) may be treated mainly by calcium channel blockers. However, in patients with INOCA, coronary functional abnormalities, including epicardial coronary spasm, reduced microvascular vasodilatation, and increased microvascular resistance, frequently coexist in various combinations. Thus, in everyday clinical practice, a combination of several types of vasodilators, such as a beta-blocker and a long-acting dihydropyridine calcium channel blocker, should constitute the second step when a single drug fails to success. In cases with refractory symptoms which seriously limit life quality, analgesic drugs or non-pharmacological interventions, including rehabilitation exercise programs, spinal cord simulation, and/or psychological treatments, might be helpful. In this section, we will discuss the treatment options for CMD, taking into consideration currently accepted pathogenic mechanisms of the disorder.

J. Takahashi · H. Shimokawa (✉)
Department of Cardiovascular Medicine, Tohoku University Graduate School of Medicine, Sendai, Miyagi, Japan
e-mail: shimo@cardio.med.tohoku.ac.jp

© Springer Nature Singapore Pte Ltd. 2021
H. Shimokawa (ed.), *Coronary Vasomotion Abnormalities*,
https://doi.org/10.1007/978-981-15-7594-5_8

Keywords Risk factor controls · Pharmacological therapy · Fasudil · Treatment algorithm

8.1 Introduction

Patients with ischemia and non-obstructive coronary artery (INOCA) often have coronary microvascular dysfunction (CMD) and are diagnosed as having microvascular angina (MVA). Recent studies demonstrated that they are at high risk for adverse cardiac events, including cardiac death, non-fatal myocardial infarction, heart failure, and hospitalization due to unstable angina [1, 2]. Nevertheless, the management of CMD represents a major unmet need because the lack of large, randomized studies involving homogeneous patient groups makes it difficult to generate evidence-based recommendations. Indeed, the guidelines of the European Society of Cardiology and the Japanese Circulation Society confirm relatively low levels of evidence for treatment of patients with CMD and no large randomized outcome trials [3, 4]. Thus, the treatment for CMD has so far been empirical because its pathophysiology appears to be multifactorial, with overlapping phenotypes that often coexist. On the other hand, recent papers have discussed the management of those patients and suggested potential therapies for CMD [5–7]. Targets for those therapies include conventional coronary risk factors and endothelial dysfunction, myocardial ischemia due to impaired coronary microvascular dilatory function or microvascular spasm, and chest pain–increased nociception [5–7]. The therapeutic aims are to improve myocardial ischemia addressing its causes, improve quality of life, and improve long-term prognosis. In this section, we will discuss the treatment options for CMD, taking into consideration currently accepted pathogenic mechanisms of the disorder.

8.2 Control of Risk Factors for Coronary Microvascular Dysfunction

The presence of CMD in patients with cardiovascular risk factors can be predictive of future development of macrovascular atherosclerosis [8]. Especially, those using intravascular ultrasound have also shown that non-obstructive coronary artery disease (CAD) is noted in a large proportion of patients with CMD [9]. Thus, aggressive management of all modifiable conventional risk factors is of paramount importance in the CMD patients [5, 10]. Smoking cessation, weight loss, adequate control of blood pressure, diabetes and metabolic abnormalities, lipid management, improved nutrition, and regular exercise may be applicable [11]. It has been demonstrated that anti-hypertensive drugs are able to improve CMD in patients with hypertension, although some differences among classes of medications may exist

[12–14]. For instance, angiotensin-converting enzyme (ACE) inhibitors and angio-tensin II receptor blockers (ARBs) have been shown to improve or even normalize endothelium-independent coronary microvascular function in hypertensive patients [12]. Furthermore, olmesartan, but not amlodipine, has been shown to improve endothelium-dependent coronary vasodilatation in hypertensive patients irrespec-tive of blood pressure (BP) reduction [13]. In contrast, another study showed that verapamil, but not enalapril, was able to improve myocardial blood flow (MBF) during atrial pacing despite a similar BP reduction [14]. These findings suggest that the favorable effects of antihypertensive drugs on CMD mainly depend on mecha-nisms other than hypotensive effect, including direct effects on vascular smooth muscle cells, an improvement of oxidative state, endothelial function, and diastolic function, as well as effects on autonomic nervous system. Statins, alone or in com-bination with ACE inhibitors, have been shown to exert beneficial effects in patients with coronary endothelial and/or vascular smooth muscle dysfunction despite non-obstructive CAD [15–17]. Unlike the cases with hypertension or hypercholesterol-emia, the effect of glycemic control on CMD in diabetic patients remains to be elucidated. Indeed, weight loss in obese patients has also been reported to improve microvascular function with increased adiponectin levels [18, 19]. Thromboxane A_2 (TXA_2) could cause microvascular constriction, platelet aggregation, and vascular injury. Thus, low-dose aspirin, which is a TXA_2 inhibitor, could provide microvas-cular protection against oxidative injury in the microcirculation [20].

CMD is also initiated by classical cardiovascular risk factors that also maintain a low-grade inflammation [21, 22]. Additionally, chronic systemic inflammation is associated with CMD possibly mediated through C-reactive protein (CRP), which levels were related to coronary flow reserve impairment in patients with a chest pain syndrome without risk factors for CAD and angiographically normal epicardial arteries [23]. Anti-inflammatory agents block associated endothelial dysfunction that plays a key role in the pathogenesis of CMD. Specific approaches to modify inflammation in CMD are difficult to assess since essentially all effective anti-ischemic and anti-atherosclerosis agents modify inflammation to some degree [24].

8.3 Pharmacological Symptomatic Therapies for Coronary Microvascular Dysfunction

8.3.1 Beta Blockers

The European Society of Cardiology guidelines for patients with MVA recommend beta-blockers as first-line and calcium channel blockers if the former are not toler-ated or efficacious [25]. Beta-blockers are able to reduce myocardial oxygen con-sumption and to improve coronary perfusion by prolonging diastolic time. In particular, beta-blocker therapy may be considered to provide therapeutic benefit for MVA patients with exercise-induced symptoms and those with increased sympathetic nervous activity as evidenced by elevated blood pressure-rate response to exercise [26, 27]. Actually, propranolol reduced the number of episodes of ST-segment depression during 24-h ECG Holter monitoring as compared to verapamil [28]. The use of atenolol has been shown to reduce the number of angina episodes and also improve the ischemic threshold [29, 30]. Carvedilol has been shown to improve endothelial function [31]. Furthermore, nebivolol, which is a highly selective beta-1 blocker with vasodilatory effects via nitric oxide (NO) production, has beneficial effects on angina and exercise capacity in patients with CMD [32]. Notably, nebivolol improved left ventricular filling pressure and coronary flow reserve (CFR) in uncomplicated arterial hypertension, suggesting the involvement of enhanced myocardial NO production and improvement of coronary microvascular function [32]. However, the effects of beta-blocker therapy on symptoms of chest pain are variable in MVA patients ranging from 19% to 60% [26]. Additionally, caution should be exercised in the use of beta-blockers in patients with microvascular spasm because they could exacerbate coronary vasoconstriction by unmasking α-adrenoceptors in the coronary circulation [5, 7].

8.3.2 Calcium Channel Blockers

Calcium channel blockers (CCBs) have potent vasodilatory effects and are therefore expected to improve the increased resistance of coronary microcirculation. However, while dihydropyridine CCBs can reduce systemic blood pressure rapidly, they might simultaneously cause a reflex increase in adrenergic activity that antagonizes their favorable vasodilatory effects. In contrast, non-dihydropyridine CCBs could decrease myocardial oxygen consumption by the negative chronotropic and inotropic effects. In a clinical setting, CCBs are widely used in patients with non-obstructive CAD and coronary vasomotor disorders including vasospastic angina (VSA). In particular, benidipine, a long-acting dihydropyridine, showed beneficial prognostic impacts in VSA patients [33]. Additionally, with the hope of improving reduced vasodilator capacity of the coronary microcirculation and reducing cardiac afterload, CCBs are often used for patients with CMD, which is supported by an experimental study showing that amlodipine improves inward remodeling in CMD [34]. In expert consensus, CCBs are likely to represent the first-line agents for patients with documented microvascular spasm or abnormal CFR and those with mainly exercise-related symptoms if beta-blockers are without effects [6, 7, 25]. However, CCBs have shown variable results in the previous trials with INOCA patients [28, 29, 35, 36]. It has been reported that intracoronary diltiazem does not improve CFR in patients with MVA [35]. Furthermore, no significant improvement in angina was noted with amlodipine in INOCA patients, [29] and verapamil failed to reduce spontaneous episodes of ischemic ST-segment changes in another study [28]. On the other hand, patients with abnormal vasodilator reserve can have improved symptoms, less nitrate use, and improved exercise tolerance with verapamil or nifedipine [36]. Moreover, long-acting nifedipine exerted cardiovascular

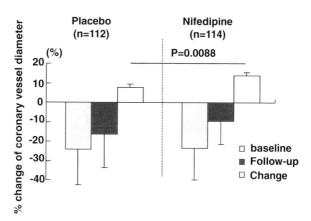

Fig. 8.1 The ENCORE II trial demonstrated that coronary vasodilator responses to intracoronary acetylcholine were improved only in the group treated with nifedipine but not in the placebo group. (Reproduced from Luscher et al. [37])

protective effects through inhibition of vascular inflammation and improvement of endothelial function in CAD patients with vasomotor dysfunction (Fig. 8.1) [37, 38]. Thus, long-acting L-type calcium channel blockers appear to be more effective for coronary microcirculation compared with short-acting ones. Importantly, it should also be noted that some patients may paradoxically experience worsening of symptoms on CCBs with a resultant withdrawal [7, 25].

8.3.3   Nitrates

Nitrates are one of the classical drugs that have been widely used for cardiovascular diseases. Nitrates act via NO signaling pathways and exert endothelium-independent vasodilatation, leading to an increase in coronary perfusion and reductions in cardiac pre- and post-load [39, 40]. With these pharmacological features, nitrates acutely improve cardiac conditions, such as angina attacks and acute heart failure. However, chronic exposure to nitrates results in a rapid development of tolerance, blunting their anti-ischemic and hemodynamic efficacy [39, 40]. Furthermore, their potential harm for cardiovascular patients, such as generation of reactive oxygen species with resultant endothelial dysfunction, [41] sympathetic nerve activation, [42] and increase in sensitivity to vasoconstrictors [43], has also been reported. Since nitrate therapy acutely improves vasospastic symptoms, [44] they are often used mainly as a concomitant therapy with CCBs in VSA patients [4, 45]. However, the effects of nitrates on the coronary microcirculation seem to be variable and rather limited. Indeed, sublingual short-acting nitrates, which are the first-line drugs to treat angina attacks in patients with MVA as well as those with obstructive CAD or epicardial spasm, were found to be effective in only about a half of patients [46]. The previous studies suggested that sublingual nitrate therapy worsened or failed to improve exercise tolerance in patients with syndrome X [47, 48]. Furthermore, chronic oral nitrate therapy with isosorbide-5-mononitrate (40 mg) also failed to improve symptoms and quality of life over a period of 4 weeks in those patients, [29] and ISDN was not helpful for patients with CMD [49]. On the basis of these results, long-acting nitrates have generally presented no positive effect and thus may not be recommended as first-line drugs for patients with CMD.

8.3.4 Nicorandil

Nicorandil has the dual properties of nitrate and K_{ATP} channel agonist, showing the cardiovascular protective effects without tolerance development [50]. This agent opens ATP-sensitive potassium channels, thereby causing dilatation of coronary resistant arterioles and possesses a nitrate moiety which dilates epicardial coronary arteries. In fact, nicorandil could cause vascular relaxation without intracellular cGMP accumulation through opening potassium channels in the plasma membrane with resultant hyperpolarization of vascular smooth muscle cells. Importantly, a functional role of K_{ATP} channels in response to nicorandil becomes more apparent when cyclic GMP formation is suppressed as in the case of nitrate tolerance [51]. A previous study demonstrated that intravenous administration of nicorandil could lead to significant improvements in scintigraphy results as well as anginal symptoms and ST-segment depression during exercise [52]. Furthermore, in another randomized placebo-controlled trial, a 2-week therapy with nicorandil in patients with microvascular angina resulted in significant improvement in exercise-induced myocardial ischemia and exercise tolerability [53]. Accordingly, where available, nicorandil should be taken into account in the treatment of patients with CMD, in particular as an alternative to nitrates.

8.3.5 ACE Inhibitors

Local tissue angiotensin II is involved in the regulation of coronary microvascular structure and function, and it also enhances the effects of sympathetic nervous system on coronary microvascular tone. Thus, renin-angiotensin system inhibition has been considered to be an appropriate therapy for patients with CMD. Furthermore, ACE inhibitors could benefit coronary vascular bed by restoring endothelial function and may improve coronary flow reserve (CFR) by bradykinin-mediated, NO-dependent mechanisms [54]. Indeed, enalapril has been demonstrated to improve CMD through increase of NO availability and reduction of oxidative stress in MVA patients [55]. It also has been demonstrated that enalapril and cilazapril reduce the magnitude of ST-segment depression and increasing the total exercise duration and time to 1 mm of ST-segment depression in MVA patients with reduced coronary flow [56, 57]. Moreover, improvements of angina symptoms and exercise capacity have been noted with the use of several kinds of ACE inhibitors [16, 58, 59]. Thus, since available studies assessing the effects of ACE inhibitors in MVA patients have generally shown beneficial results, more proactive use of the agents should be recommended in patients with CMD.

8.3.6 Ranolazine

Ranolazine is an anti-ischemic dug that acts via inhibiting the transmembrane late sodium current, resulting in reduction of intracellular calcium levels and prevention of calcium overload during ischemia [60]. Thus, ranolazine is considered to be able to improve myocardial relaxation and left ventricular diastolic function [60]. The effect of ranolazine on CMD has been conflicting in the pilot placebo-controlled trials, [61, 62] whereas a recent large randomized crossover trial of ranolazine vs. placebo found no difference in symptoms or cardiac magnetic resonance imaging-myocardial perfusion reserve [63]. However, in a pre-defined subgroup who had CFR assessed invasively, symptomatic patients with CFR <2.5 and non-obstructive CAD showed improved angina and myocardial perfusion with ranolazine, indicating that ranolazine provides a promising management option for patients with CMD and low CFR [64].

8.3.7 Ivabradine

Selective If-channel blockade using ivabradine is a specific bradycardic agent that selectively reduces sinus node activity through inhibition of the If current [65]. In contrast to β-blockers, ivabradine does not cause vasoconstriction or negative inotropic effects [65]. Beneficial effects of ivabradine in IHD are mediated by its indirect effects to improve exercise tolerance, prolong time to ischemia during exercise, and reduce angina severity and frequency compared with other antianginal agents in patients with stable angina [65, 66]. Ivabradine improved angina in patients with MVA but coronary microvascular function did not change, suggesting that symptomatic improvement could be attributed to heart-rate-lowering effect [62]. However, others have found that ivabradine improves CFR in non-obstructed coronary arteries of patients with stable CAD at both baseline and paced heart rates identical to that before treatment [67]. Thus, ivabradine may improve CFR in patients with stable CAD. These effects persist even after heart rate correction, indicating improved microvascular function [68]. Thus, it is possible that ivabradine and/or perhaps some other If-channel inhibitors have a role in CMD patients, although further studies are needed.

8.3.8 Xanthine Antagonists

Xanthine derivatives are considered to have favorable effects on nociception in MVA patients. They were suggested to have analgesic effects that result from antagonizing stimulation of cardiac nerve pain fibers through adenosine, a major mediator of ischemic chest pain [69]. They may also have anti-ischemic actions through attenuation of the coronary microvascular steal phenomenon observed in MVA patients [70]. Aminophylline may improve exercise tolerance and exercise-induced myocardial ischemia in patients with INOCA [71, 72]. Clinically, these drugs represent a bailout option in completely refractory patients before more invasive methods such as spinal cord stimulation may be considered.

8.4 Expectation for Rho-Kinase Inhibitor, Fasudil, as a Therapeutic Option for CMD

Enhanced Rho-kinase activity plays important roles in the pathogenesis of both epicardial coronary and microvascular spasm [73]. In particular, the pathogenetic mechanisms of CMD appear to be heterogeneous, and many confounding cardiovascular risk factors cause both endothelial dysfunction and VSMC hyperconstriction, where activated Rho-kinase pathway plays important roles (Fig. 8.2). Furthermore, Rho-kinase pathway has also been shown to be substantially involved in inflammatory cell accumulation in blood vessel adventitia, [74] and a pathogenetic mechanism in patients with chest pain and non-obstructive CAD [75]. Rho-kinase enhances myosin light chain phosphorylation through inhibition of myosin-binding subunit of myosin phosphatase, leading to vascular smooth muscle hypercontraction (Fig. 8.3) [76]. Fasudil, a specific Rho-kinase inhibitor, is highly effective in preventing acetylcholine-induced coronary spasm and resultant myocardial ischemia (Fig. 8.3) [77]. Indeed, intracoronary fasudil is effective not only for patients with epicardial coronary spasm [77] but also for approximately two thirds of MVA patients [78]. Specifically in the latter, Mohri et al. studied consecutive 18 patients with angina and normal epicardial coronaries in whom intracoronary ACh induced myocardial ischemia (defined as ischemic electrocardiographic changes,

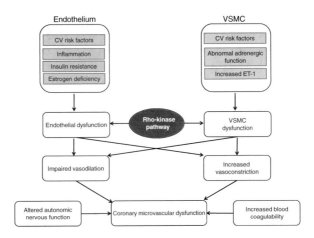

Fig. 8.2 Pathogenesis of coronary microvascular dysfunction and important role of Rho-kinase in it. The pathogenetic mechanisms of coronary microvascular dysfunction appear to be heterogeneous, and many confounding cardiovascular risk factors cause both endothelial dysfunction and VSMC hyperconstriction, where activated Rho-kinase pathway may play an important role. *CV* cardiovascular, *ET-1* endothelin-1

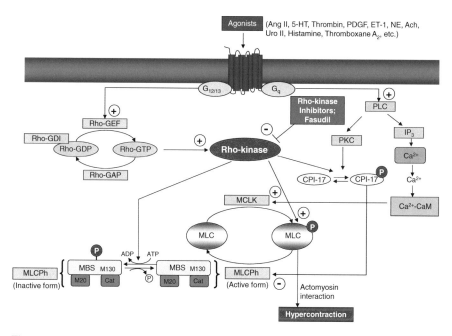

Fig. 8.3 Roles of the Rho/Rho-kinase signaling pathway in VSMC hyperconstriction. Contraction is induced by increased phosphorylation of MLC. The agonist-induced activation of G-protein-coupled receptors leads to the stimulation of MLCK through an increase in intracellular Ca^{2+} concentration and inhibition of MLCPh. Following stimulation by various agonists, the Rho/Rho-kinase-mediated pathway is activated, resulting in the inhibition of MLCPh (through phosphorylation of its MBS), with a resultant increase in MLC phosphorylation. This Rho-kinase-mediated contraction of VSMC can occur independently of intracellular Ca^{2+} levels and is known as "calcium sensitization." Rho-kinase can also increase MLC phosphorylation and contractility by inactivating MLCPh after phosphorylation of CPI-17 or by direct phosphorylation of MLC. *ACh* acetylcholine, *Ang II* angiotensin II, *Cat* catalytic subunit, *ET-1* endothelin-1, *IP₃* inositol (1,4,5)-trisphosphate, *M20* 20-kDa subunit, *NE* norepinephrine, *PLC* phospholipase C, *PDGF* platelet-derived growth factor, *Uro II* urotensin II. Stimulation is denoted by +; inhibition is denoted by −. (Reproduced from Shimokawa et al. [76])

myocardial lactate production, or both) without angiographically demonstrable epicardial coronary vasospasm. All patients underwent a second ACh challenge test after pretreatment with either saline ($n = 5$) or fasudil (4.5 mg intracoronarily, $n = 13$). While myocardial ischemia was reproducibly induced by ACh in the saline group, 11 of the 13 patients pretreated with fasudil had no evidence of myocardial ischemia during the second infusion of ACh ($P < 0.01$). The lactate extraction ratio (median value [interquartile range]) during ACh infusion was improved by fasudil pretreatment, from −0.16 (−0.25 to 0.04) to 0.09 (0.05 to 0.18) ($P = 0.0125$) (Fig. 8.4). These results strongly indicate that fasudil is able to ameliorate myocardial ischemia in patients who were most likely having coronary microvascular spasm. Furthermore, Fukumoto et al. examined whether Rho-kinase is involved in coronary microvascular constriction in patients with obstructive CAD [79]. In brief, intracoronary administration of fasudil (300 mg/min for 15 min) significantly increased oxygen saturation in coronary sinus vein from 37 ± 3% to

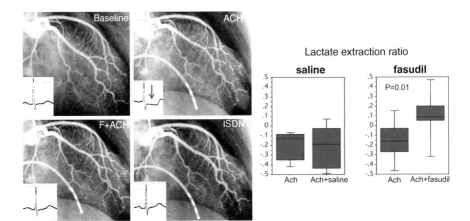

Fig. 8.4 Clinical findings in a patient with microvascular angina. Representative coronary angiography and ECG recordings (left) and group data comparison of the lactate extraction ratio during acetylcholine (ACh) infusion with ($n = 13$, fasudil group) and without pre-treatment of fasudil ($n = 5$, saline group) (right). Intracoronary administration of ACh caused no appreciable vasoconstriction of epicardial coronary arteries, whereas ECG changes and myocardial lactate production indicated the occurrence of myocardial ischemia. Intracoronary pre-treatment with fasudil abolished the ACh-induced myocardial ischemia. *F* fasudil, *ISDN* isosorbidedinitrate. (Reproduced from Masumoto et al. [77])

$41 \pm 3\%$ ($P < 0.05$) but not in six age-matched controls (from $42 \pm 3\%$ to $43 \pm 3\%$, P=NS). Importantly, intracoronary fasudil significantly ameliorated pacing-induced myocardial ischemia in patients with obstructive CAD (magnitudes of symptom, 1.5 ± 0.6 to 0.6 ± 0.4, $P < 0.01$; ischemic ST-segment depression, 1.8 ± 0.3 to 1.0 ± 0.2 mm, $P < 0.01$; percent lactate production, $50 \pm 17\%$ to $0.4 \pm 7\%$, $P < 0.01$) without significant hemodynamic changes [78]. These results provide the evidence that Rho-kinase is substantially involved in the pathogenesis of CMD associated with myocardial ischemia in patients with obstructive CAD, suggesting that fasudil could be a therapeutic option for CMD with obstructive CAD. Myocardial hypertrophy induced by pressure overload leads to myocardial dysfunction, CMD, and ischemia possibly due to oxidative stress, enhanced vasoconstriction to endothelin-1, and compromised endothelial NO function via elevated Rho-kinase signaling [80]. Fasudil may be effective in a wide variety of CMD where Rho-kinase plays an important role.

8.5   A Rational Approach for the Management of CMD Patients

Considering the results of the CorMicA trial, [81] the latest ESC guidelines state that treatment of microvascular angina should address the dominant mechanism of microcirculatory dysfunction (Fig. 8.5). In patients with impaired microcirculatory conductance with abnormal CFR <2.0 or IMR ≥25 units, and a negative acetylcholine provocation test, beta-blockers, ACE inhibitors, and statins, along with lifestyle modifications and weight loss, are indicated. On the other hand, patients developing ECG changes and angina in response to acetyl-choline testing but without severe epicardial vasoconstriction (all suggestive of microvascular spasm) may be treated mainly by CCBs like VSA patients. However, as demonstrated by our group, in patients with INOCA, coronary functional abnormalities, including epicardial coronary spasm, reduced micro-vascular vasodilatation, and increased microvascular resistance, frequently coexist in various combinations [75]. Thus, in everyday clinical practice, the first-line medication is represented by beta-blockers or long-acting dihydro-pyridine CCBs, while a combination of them should constitute the second step when single drugs fail to success. In some cases, long-acting nitrates could be added, although there is less evidence of their actual efficacy. A proposed treat-ment algorithm for patients with MVA is shown in Fig. 8.5. All patients should receive optical risk control. If symptoms are not well controlled, addition of traditional and non-traditional anti-ischemic drugs is recommended. Ivabradine can be added when beta-blockers are scarcely tolerated, while ranolazine should be considered in MVA patients with reduced CFR. In cases with refractory symptoms that seriously limit quality of life, analgesic drugs or non-pharmaco-logical interventions including rehabilitation exercise programs, spinal cord simulation, psychological treatments, and shock wave therapy [82] might be helpful.

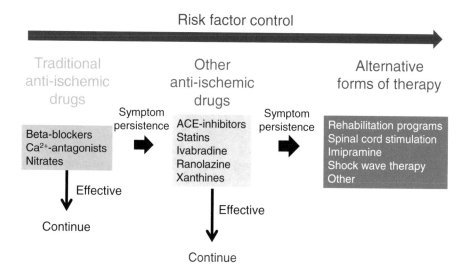

Fig. 8.5 Treatment algorithm for patients with microvascular angina

References

1. Pepine CJ, Anderson RD, Sharaf BL, Reis SE, Smith KM, Handberg EM, Johnson BD, Sopko G, Bairey Merz CN. Coronary microvascular reactivity to adenosine predicts adverse outcome in women evaluated for suspected ischemia results from the National Heart, Lung and Blood Institute WISE (women's ischemia syndrome evaluation) study. J Am Coll Cardiol. 2010;55(25):2825–32. https://doi.org/10.1016/j.jacc.2010.01.054.
2. Lin FY, Shaw LJ, Dunning AM, Labounty TM, Choi JH, Weinsaft JW, Koduru S, Gomez MJ, Delago AJ, Callister TQ, Berman DS, Min JK. Mortality risk in symptomatic patients with nonobstructive coronary artery disease: a prospective 2-center study of 2,583 patients undergoing 64-detector row coronary computed tomographic angiography. J Am Coll Cardiol. 2011;58(5):510–9. https://doi.org/10.1016/j.jacc.2010.11.078.
3. Knuuti J, Wijns W, Saraste A, Capodanno D, Barbato E, Funck-Brentano C, Prescott E, Storey RF, Deaton C, Cuisset T, Agewall S, Dickstein K, Edvardsen T, Escaned J, Gersh BJ, Svitil P, Gilard M, Hasdai D, Hatala R, Mahfoud F, Masip J, Muneretto C, Valgimigli M, Achenbach S, Bax JJ. 2019 ESC guidelines for the diagnosis and management of chronic coronary syndromes. Eur Heart J. 2020;41(3):407–77. https://doi.org/10.1093/eurheartj/ehz425.
4. JCS Joint Working Group. Guidelines for diagnosis and treatment of patients with vasospastic angina (coronary spastic angina) (JCS 2013). Circ J. 2014;78(11):2779–801. https://doi.org/10.1253/circj.cj-66-0098.
5. Lim TK, Choy AJ, Khan F, Belch JJ, Struthers AD, Lang CC. Therapeutic development in cardiac syndrome X: a need to target the underlying pathophysiology. Cardiovasc Ther. 2009;27(1):49–58. https://doi.org/10.1111/j.1755-5922.2008.00070.x.
6. Bairey Merz CN, Pepine CJ, Walsh MN, Fleg JL. Ischemia and no obstructive coronary artery disease (INOCA): developing evidence-based therapies and research agenda for the next decade. Circulation. 2017;135(11):1075–92. https://doi.org/10.1161/CIRCULATIONAHA.116.024534.
7. Bairey Merz CN, Pepine CJ, Shimokawa H, Berry C. Treatment of coronary microvascular dysfunction. Cardiovasc Res. 2020;116(4):856–70. https://doi.org/10.1093/cvr/cvaa006.
8. Pirat B, Bozbas H, Simsek V, Yildirir A, Sade LE, Gursoy Y, Altin C, Atar I, Muderrisoglu H. Impaired coronary flow reserve in patients with metabolic syndrome. Atherosclerosis. 2008;201(1):112–6. https://doi.org/10.1016/j.atherosclerosis.2008.02.016.
9. Khuddus MA, Pepine CJ, Handberg EM, Bairey Merz CN, Sopko G, Bavry AA, Denardo SJ, McGorray SP, Smith KM, Sharaf BL, Nicholls SJ, Nissen SE, Anderson RD. An intravascular ultrasound analysis in women experiencing chest pain in the absence of obstructive coronary artery disease: a substudy from the National Heart, Lung and Blood Institute-sponsored women's ischemia syndrome evaluation (WISE). J Interv Cardiol. 2010;23(6):511–9. https://doi.org/10.1111/j.1540-8183.2010.00598.x.
10. Stampfer MJ, Hu FB, Manson JE, Rimm EB, Willett WC. Primary prevention of coronary heart disease in women through diet and lifestyle. N Engl J Med. 2000;343(1):16–22. https://doi.org/10.1056/NEJM200007063430103.
11. Eriksson BE, Tyni-Lenne R, Svedenhag J, Hallin R, Jensen-Urstad K, Jensen-Urstad M, Bergman K, Selvén C. Physical training in syndrome X: physical training counteracts deconditioning and pain in syndrome X. J Am Coll Cardiol. 2000;36(5):1619–25. https://doi.org/10.1016/s0735-1097(00)00931-1.
12. Motz W, Strauer BE. Improvement of coronary flow reserve after long-term therapy with enalapril. Hypertension. 1996;27(5):1031–8. https://doi.org/10.1161/01.hyp.27.5.1031.
13. Naya M, Tsukamoto T, Morita K, Katoh C, Furumoto T, Fujii S, Tamaki N, Tsutsui H. Olmesartan, but not amlodipine, improves endothelium-dependent coronary dilation in hypertensive patients. J Am Coll Cardiol. 2007;50(12):1144–9. https://doi.org/10.1016/j.jacc.2007.06.013.
14. Brush JE Jr, Cannon RO 3rd, Schenke WH, Bonow RO, Leon MB, Maron BJ, Epstein SE. Angina due to coronary microvascular disease in hypertensive patients without left

ventricular hypertrophy. N Engl J Med. 1988;319(20):1302–7. https://doi.org/10.1056/NEJM198811173192002.

15. Caliskan M, Erdogan D, Gullu H, Topcu S, Ciftci O, Yildirir A, Muderrisoglu H. Effects of atorvastatin on coronary flow reserve in patients with slow coronary flow. Clin Cardiol. 2007;30(9):475–9. https://doi.org/10.1002/clc.20140.

16. Pizzi C, Manfrini O, Fontana F, Bugiardini R. Angiotensin-converting enzyme inhibitors and 3-hydroxy-3-methylglutaryl coenzyme A reductase in cardiac syndrome X: role of superoxide dismutase activity. Circulation. 2004;109(1):53–8. https://doi.org/10.1161/01.CIR.0000100722.34034.E4.

17. Guethlin M, Kasel AM, Coppenrath K, Ziegler S, Delius W, Schwaiger M. Delayed response of myocardial flow reserve to lipid-lowering therapy with fluvastatin. Circulation. 1999;99(4):475–81. https://doi.org/10.1161/01.cir.99.4.475.

18. Nerla R, Tarzia P, Sestito A, Di Monaco A, Infusino F, Matera D, Greco F, Tacchino RM, Lanza GA, Crea F. Effect of bariatric surgery on peripheral flow-mediated dilation and coronary microvascular function. Nutr Metab Cardiovasc Dis. 2012;22(8):626–34. https://doi.org/10.1016/j.numecd.2010.10.004.

19. Quercioli A, Montecucco F, Pataky Z, Thomas A, Ambrosio G, Staub C, Di Marzo V, Ratib O, Mach F, Golay A, Schindler TH. Improvement in coronary circulatory function in morbidly obese individuals after gastric bypass-induced weight loss: relation to alterations in endocannabinoids and adipocytokines. Eur Heart J. 2013;34(27):2063–73. https://doi.org/10.1093/eurheartj/eht085.

20. Chiang CY, Chien CY, Qiou WY, Chang C, Yu IS, Chang PY, Chien CT. Genetic depletion of thromboxane A2/thromboxane-prostanoid receptor signalling prevents microvascular dysfunction in ischaemia/reperfusion injury. Thromb Haemost. 2018;118(11):1982–96. https://doi.org/10.1055/s-0038-1672206.

21. Granger DN, Rodrigues SF, Yildirim A, Senchenkova EY. Microvascular responses to cardiovascular risk factors. Microcirculation. 2010;17(3):192–205. https://doi.org/10.1111/j.1549-8719.2009.00015.x.

22. Herrmann J, Kaski JC, Lerman A. Coronary microvascular dysfunction in the clinical setting: from mystery to reality. Eur Heart J. 2012;33(22):2771–82b. https://doi.org/10.1093/eurheartj/ehs246.

23. Recio-Mayoral A, Mason JC, Kaski JC, Rubens MB, Harari OA, Camici PG. Chronic inflammation and coronary microvascular dysfunction in patients without risk factors for coronary artery disease. Eur Heart J. 2009;30(15):1837–43. https://doi.org/10.1093/eurheartj/ehp205.

24. Lucas AR, Korol R, Pepine CJ. Inflammation in atherosclerosis: some thoughts about acute coronary syndromes. Circulation. 2006;113(17):e728–32. https://doi.org/10.1161/CIRCULATIONAHA.105.601492.

25. Task Force Members, Montalescot G, Sechtem U, Achenbach S, Andreotti F, Arden C, Budaj A, Bugiardini R, Crea F, Cuisset T, DiMario C, Ferreira R, Gersh BJ, Gitt AK, Hulot JS, Marx N, Opie LH, Pfisterer M, Prescott E, Ruschitzka F, Sabate M, Senior R, Taggart DP, van der Wall EE, CJM V. 2013 ESC guidelines on the management of stable coronary artery disease: the Task Force on the management of stable coronary artery disease of the European Society of Cardiology. Eur Heart J. 2013;34(38):2949–3003. https://doi.org/10.1093/eurheartj/eht296.

26. Kaski JC, Valenzuela Garcia LF. Therapeutic options for the management of patients with cardiac syndrome X. Eur Heart J. 2001;22(4):283–93. https://doi.org/10.1053/euhj.2000.2152.

27. Fragasso G, Chierchia SL, Pizzetti G, Rossetti E, Carlino M, Gerosa S, Carandente O, Fedele A, Cattaneo N. Impaired left ventricular filling dynamics in patients with angina and angiographically normal coronary arteries: effect of beta adrenergic blockade. Heart. 1997;77(1):32–9. https://doi.org/10.1136/hrt.77.1.32.

28. Bugiardini R, Borghi A, Biagetti L, Puddu P. Comparison of verapamil versus propranolol therapy in syndrome X. Am J Cardiol. 1989;63(5):286–90. https://doi.org/10.1016/0002-9149(89)90332-9.

29. Lanza GA, Colonna G, Pasceri V, Maseri A. Atenolol versus amlodipine versus isosorbide-5-mononitrate on anginal symptoms in syndrome X. Am J Cardiol. 1999;84(7):854–6., A8. https://doi.org/10.1016/s0002-9149(99)00450-6.

30. Leonardo F, Fragasso G, Rossetti E, Dabrowski P, Pagnotta P, Rosano GM, Chierchia SL. Comparison of trimetazidine with atenolol in patients with syndrome X: effects on diastolic function and exercise tolerance. Cardiologia. 1999;44(12):1065–9.

31. Matsuda Y, Akita H, Terashima M, Shiga N, Kanazawa K, Yokoyama M. Carvedilol improves endothelium-dependent dilatation in patients with coronary artery disease. Am Heart J. 2000;140(5):753–9. https://doi.org/10.1067/mhj.2000.110093.

32. Togni M, Vigorito F, Windecker S, Abrecht L, Wenaweser P, Cook S, Billinger M, Meier B, Hess OM. Does the beta-blocker nebivolol increase coronary flow reserve? Cardiovasc Drugs Ther. 2007;21(2):99–108. https://doi.org/10.1007/s10557-006-0494-7.

33. Nishigaki K, Inoue Y, Yamanouchi Y, Fukumoto Y, Yasuda S, Sueda S, Urata H, Shimokawa H, Minatoguchi S. Prognostic effects of calcium channel blockers in patients with vasospastic angina—a meta-analysis. Circ J. 2010;74(9):1943–50. https://doi.org/10.1253/circj.cj-10-0292.

34. Sorop O, Bakker EN, Pistea A, Spaan JA, VanBavel E. Calcium channel blockade prevents pressure-dependent inward remodeling in isolated subendocardial resistance vessels. Am J Physiol Heart Circ Physiol. 2006;291(3):H1236–45. https://doi.org/10.1152/ajpheart.00838.2005.

35. Sutsch G, Oechslin E, Mayer I, Hess OM. Effect of diltiazem on coronary flow reserve in patients with microvascular angina. Int J Cardiol. 1995;52(2):135–43. https://doi.org/10.1016/0167-5273(95)02458-9.

36. Cannon RO 3rd, Watson RM, Rosing DR, Epstein SE. Efficacy of calcium channel blocker therapy for angina pectoris resulting from small-vessel coronary artery disease and abnormal vasodilator reserve. Am J Cardiol. 1985;56(4):242–6. https://doi.org/10.1016/0002-9149(85)90842-2.

37. Luscher TF, Pieper M, Tendera M, Vrolix M, Rutsch W, van den Branden F, Gil R, Bischoff KO, Haude M, Fischer D, Meinertz T, Münzel T. A randomized placebo-controlled study on the effect of nifedipine on coronary endothelial function and plaque formation in patients with coronary artery disease: the ENCORE II study. Eur Heart J. 2009;30(13):1590–7. https://doi.org/10.1093/eurheartj/ehp151.

38. Tsuburaya R, Takahashi J, Nakamura A, Nozaki E, Sugi M, Yamamoto Y, Hiramoto T, Horiguchi S, Inoue K, Goto T, Kato A, Shinozaki T, Ishida E, Miyata S, Yasuda S, Shimokawa H, NOVEL Investigators. Beneficial effects of long-acting nifedipine on coronary vasomotion abnormalities after drug-eluting stent implantation: the NOVEL study. Eur Heart J. 2016;37(35):2713–21. https://doi.org/10.1093/eurheartj/ehw256.

39. Munzel T, Daiber A, Gori T. More answers to the still unresolved question of nitrate tolerance. Eur Heart J. 2013;34(34):2666–73. https://doi.org/10.1093/eurheartj/eht249.

40. Daiber A, Wenzel P, Oelze M, Munzel T. New insights into bioactivation of organic nitrates, nitrate tolerance and cross-tolerance. Clin Res Cardiol. 2008;97(1):12–20. https://doi.org/10.1007/s00392-007-0588-7.

41. Thomas GR, DiFabio JM, Gori T, Parker JD. Once daily therapy with isosorbide-5-mononitrate causes endothelial dysfunction in humans: evidence of a free-radical-mediated mechanism. J Am Coll Cardiol. 2007;49(12):1289–95. https://doi.org/10.1016/j.jacc.2006.10.074.

42. Gori T, Floras JS, Parker JD. Effects of nitroglycerin treatment on baroreflex sensitivity and short-term heart rate variability in humans. J Am Coll Cardiol. 2002;40(11):2000–5. https://doi.org/10.1016/s0735-1097(02)02532-9.

43. Heitzer T, Just H, Brockhoff C, Meinertz T, Olschewski M, Munzel T. Long-term nitroglycerin treatment is associated with supersensitivity to vasoconstrictors in men with stable coronary artery disease: prevention by concomitant treatment with captopril. J Am Coll Cardiol. 1998;31(1):83–8. https://doi.org/10.1016/s0735-1097(97)00431-2.

44. Rizzon P, Scrutinio D, Mangini SG, Lagioia R, de Toma L. Randomized placebo-controlled comparative study of nifedipine, verapamil and isosorbide dinitrate in the treatment of angina

at rest. Eur Heart J. 1986;7(1):67–76. https://doi.org/10.1093/oxfordjournals.eurheartj. a061960.

45. Takahashi J, Nihei T, Takagi Y, Miyata S, Odaka Y, Tsunoda R, Seki A, Sumiyoshi T, Matsui M, Goto T, Tanabe Y, Sueda S, Momomura S, Yasuda S, Ogawa H, Shimokawa H, Japanese Coronary Spasm Association. Prognostic impact of chronic nitrate therapy in patients with vasospastic angina: multicentre registry study of the Japanese Coronary Spasm Association. Eur Heart J. 2015;36(4):228–37. https://doi.org/10.1093/eurheartj/ehu313.

46. Kaski JC, Rosano GM, Collins P, Nihoyannopoulos P, Maseri A, Poole-Wilson PA. Cardiac syndrome X: clinical characteristics and left ventricular function. Long-term follow-up study. J Am Coll Cardiol. 1995;25(4):807–14. https://doi.org/10.1016/0735-1097(94)00507-M.

47. Radice M, Giudici V, Pusineri E, Breghi L, Nicoli T, Peci P, Giani P, De Ambroggi L. Different effects of acute administration of aminophylline and nitroglycerin on exercise capacity in patients with syndrome X. Am J Cardiol. 1996;78(1):88–92. https://doi.org/10.1016/s0002-9149(96)00231-7.

48. Lanza GA, Manzoli A, Bia E, Crea F, Maseri A. Acute effects of nitrates on exercise testing in patients with syndrome X. Clinical and pathophysiological implications. Circulation. 1994;90(6):2695–700. https://doi.org/10.1161/01.cir.90.6.2695.

49. Russo G, Di Franco A, Lamendola P, Tarzia P, Nerla R, Stazi A, Villano A, Sestito A, Lanza GA, Crea F. Lack of effect of nitrates on exercise stress test results in patients with microvascular angina. Cardiovasc Drugs Ther. 2013;27(3):229–34. https://doi.org/10.1007/s10557-013-6439-z.

50. Horinaka S. Use of nicorandil in cardiovascular disease and its optimization. Drugs. 2011;71(9):1105–19. https://doi.org/10.2165/11592300-000000000-00000.

51. O'Rourke ST. K_{ATP} channel activation mediates nicorandil-induced relaxation of nitratetolerant coronary arteries. J Cardiovasc Pharmacol. 1996;27(6):831–7. https://doi.org/10.1097/00005344-199606000-00010.

52. Yamabe H, Namura H, Yano T, Fujita H, Kim S, Iwahashi M, Maeda K, Yokoyama M. Effect of nicorandil on abnormal coronary flow reserve assessed by exercise 201Tl scintigraphy in patients with angina pectoris and nearly normal coronary arteriograms. Cardiovasc Drugs Ther. 1995;9(6):755–61. https://doi.org/10.1007/bf00879868.

53. Chen JW, Lee WL, Hsu NW, Lin SJ, Ting CT, Wang SP, Chang MS. Effects of short-term treatment of nicorandil on exercise-induced myocardial ischemia and abnormal cardiac autonomic activity in microvascular angina. Am J Cardiol. 1997;80(1):32–8. https://doi.org/10.1016/s0002-9149(97)00279-8.

54. Nikolaidis LA, Doverspike A, Huerbin R, Hentosz T, Shannon RP. Angiotensin-converting enzyme inhibitors improve coronary flow reserve in dilated cardiomyopathy by a bradykinin-mediated, nitric oxide-dependent mechanism. Circulation. 2002;105(23):2785–90. https://doi.org/10.1161/01.cir.0000017433.90061.2e.

55. Camici PG, Marraccini P, Gistri R, Salvadori PA, Sorace O, L'Abbate A. Adrenergically mediated coronary vasoconstriction in patients with syndrome X. Cardiovasc Drugs Ther. 1994;8(2):221–6. https://doi.org/10.1007/bf00877330.

56. Kaski JC, Rosano G, Gavrielides S, Chen L. Effects of angiotensin-converting enzyme inhibition on exercise-induced angina and ST segment depression in patients with microvascular angina. J Am Coll Cardiol. 1994;23(3):652–7. https://doi.org/10.1016/0735-1097(94)90750-1.

57. Nalbantgil I, Onder R, Altintig A, Nalbantgil S, Kiliccioglu B, Boydak B, Yilmaz H. Therapeutic benefits of cilazapril in patients with syndrome X. Cardiology. 1998;89(2):130–3. https://doi.org/10.1159/000006768.

58. Chen JW, Hsu NW, Wu TC, Lin SJ, Chang MS. Long-term angiotensin-converting enzyme inhibition reduces plasma asymmetric dimethylarginine and improves endothelial nitric oxide bioavailability and coronary microvascular function in patients with syndrome X. Am J Cardiol. 2002;90(9):974–82. https://doi.org/10.1016/s0002-9149(02)02664-4.

59. Pauly DF, Johnson BD, Anderson RD, Handberg EM, Smith KM, Cooper-DeHoff RM, Sopko G, Sharaf BM, Kelsey SF, Merz CN, Pepine CJ. In women with symptoms of cardiac ischemia,

nonobstructive coronary arteries, and microvascular dysfunction, angiotensin-converting enzyme inhibition is associated with improved microvascular function: a double-blind randomized study from the National Heart, Lung and Blood Institute women's ischemia syndrome evaluation (WISE). Am Heart J. 2011;162(4):678–84. https://doi.org/10.1016/j.ahj.2011.07.011.

60. Hasenfuss G, Maier LS. Mechanism of action of the new anti-ischemia drug ranolazine. Clin Res Cardiol. 2008;97(4):222–6. https://doi.org/10.1007/s00392-007-0612-y.

61. Mehta PK, Goykhman P, Thomson LE, Shufelt C, Wei J, Yang Y, Gill E, Minissian M, Shaw LJ, Slomka PJ, Slivka M, Berman DS, Bairey Merz CN. Ranolazine improves angina in women with evidence of myocardial ischemia but no obstructive coronary artery disease. JACC Cardiovasc Imaging. 2011;4(5):514–22. https://doi.org/10.1016/j.jcmg.2011.03.007.

62. Villano A, Di Franco A, Nerla R, Sestito A, Tarzia P, Lamendola P, Di Monaco A, Sarullo FM, Lanza GA, Crea F. Effects of ivabradine and ranolazine in patients with microvascular angina pectoris. Am J Cardiol. 2013;112(1):8–13. https://doi.org/10.1016/j.amjcard.2013.02.045.

63. Bairey Merz CN, Handberg EM, Shufelt CL, Mehta PK, Minissian MB, Wei J, Thomson LE, Berman DS, Shaw LJ, Petersen JW, Brown GH, Anderson RD, Shuster JJ, Cook-Wiens G, Rogatko A, Pepine CJ. A randomized, placebo-controlled trial of late Na current inhibition (ranolazine) in coronary microvascular dysfunction (CMD): impact on angina and myocardial perfusion reserve. Eur Heart J. 2016;37(19):1504–13. https://doi.org/10.1093/eurheartj/ehv647.

64. Rambarat CA, Elgendy IY, Handberg EM, Bairey Merz CN, Wei J, Minissian MB, Nelson MD, Thomson LEJ, Berman DS, Shaw LJ, Cook-Wiens G, Pepine CJ. Late sodium channel blockade improves angina and myocardial perfusion in patients with severe coronary microvascular dysfunction: women's ischemia syndrome evaluation-coronary vascular dysfunction ancillary study. Int J Cardiol. 2019;276:8–13. https://doi.org/10.1016/j.ijcard.2018.09.081.

65. Borer JS, Fox K, Jaillon P, Lerebours G, Ivabradine IG. Antianginal and antiischemic effects of ivabradine, an I(f) inhibitor, in stable angina: a randomized, double-blind, multicentered, placebo-controlled trial. Circulation. 2003;107(6):817–23. https://doi.org/10.1161/01.cir.0000048143.25023.87.

66. Tardif JC, Ford I, Tendera M, Bourassa MG, Fox K, Investigators I. Efficacy of ivabradine, a new selective I(f) inhibitor, compared with atenolol in patients with chronic stable angina. Eur Heart J. 2005;26(23):2529–36. https://doi.org/10.1093/eurheartj/ehi586.

67. Skalidis EI, Hamilos MI, Chlouverakis G, Zacharis EA, Vardas PE. Ivabradine improves coronary flow reserve in patients with stable coronary artery disease. Atherosclerosis. 2011;215(1):160–5. https://doi.org/10.1016/j.atherosclerosis.2010.11.035.

68. Camici PG, Gloekler S, Levy BI, Skalidis E, Tagliamonte E, Vardas P, Heusch G. Ivabradine in chronic stable angina: effects by and beyond heart rate reduction. Int J Cardiol. 2016;215:1–6. https://doi.org/10.1016/j.ijcard.2016.04.001.

69. Crea F, Pupita G, Galassi AR, el-Tamimi H, Kaski JC, Davies G, Maseri A. Role of adenosine in pathogenesis of anginal pain. Circulation. 1990;81(1):164–72. https://doi.org/10.1161/01.cir.81.1.164.

70. Crea F, Gaspardone A, Araujo L, Da Silva R, Kaski JC, Davies G, Maseri A. Effects of aminophylline on cardiac function and regional myocardial perfusion: implications regarding its antiischemic action. Am Heart J. 1994;127(4 Pt 1):817–24. https://doi.org/10.1016/0002-8703(94)90548-7.

71. Elliott PM, Krzyzowska-Dickinson K, Calvino R, Hann C, Kaski JC. Effect of oral aminophylline in patients with angina and normal coronary arteriograms (cardiac syndrome X). Heart. 1997;77(6):523–6. https://doi.org/10.1136/hrt.77.6.523.

72. Yoshio H, Shimizu M, Kita Y, Ino H, Kaku B, Taki J, Takeda R. Effects of short-term aminophylline administration on cardiac functional reserve in patients with syndrome X. J Am Coll Cardiol. 1995;25(7):1547–51. https://doi.org/10.1016/0735-1097(95)00097-n.

73. Shimokawa H. 2014 Williams Harvey lecture: importance of coronary vasomotion abnormalities-from bench to bedside. Eur Heart J. 2014;35(45):3180–93. https://doi.org/10.1093/eurheartj/ehu427.

74. Ohyama K, Matsumoto Y, Takanami K, Ota H, Nishimiya K, Sugisawa J, Tsuchiya S, Amamizu H, Uzuka H, Suda A, Shindo T, Kikuchi Y, Hao K, Tsuburaya R, Takahashi J, Miyata S, Sakata Y, Takase K, Shimokawa H. Coronary adventitial and perivascular adipose tissue inflammation in patients with vasospastic angina. J Am Coll Cardiol. 2018;71(4):414–25. https://doi.org/10.1016/j.jacc.2017.11.046.

75. Suda A, Takahashi J, Hao K, Kikuchi Y, Shindo T, Ikeda S, Sato K, Sugisawa J, Matsumoto Y, Miyata S, Sakata Y, Shimokawa H. Coronary functional abnormalities in patients with angina and nonobstructive coronary artery disease. J Am Coll Cardiol. 2019;74(19):2350–60. https://doi.org/10.1016/j.jacc.2019.08.1056.

76. Shimokawa H, Sunamura S, Satoh K. RhoA/Rho-kinase in the cardiovascular system. Circ Res. 2016;118(2):352–66. https://doi.org/10.1161/CIRCRESAHA.115.306532.

77. Masumoto A, Mohri M, Shimokawa H, Urakami L, Usui M, Takeshita A. Suppression of coronary artery spasm by the Rho-kinase inhibitor fasudil in patients with vasospastic angina. Circulation. 2002;105(13):1545–7. https://doi.org/10.1161/hc1002.105938.

78. Mohri M, Shimokawa H, Hirakawa Y, Masumoto A, Takeshita A. Rho-kinase inhibition with intracoronary fasudil prevents myocardial ischemia in patients with coronary microvascular spasm. J Am Coll Cardiol. 2003;41(1):15–9. https://doi.org/10.1016/s0735-1097(02)02632-3.

79. Fukumoto Y, Matoba T, Ito A, Tanaka H, Kishi T, Hayashidani S, Abe K, Takeshita A, Shimokawa H. Acute vasodilator effects of a Rho-kinase inhibitor, fasudil, in patients with severe pulmonary hypertension. Heart. 2005;91(3):391–2. https://doi.org/10.1136/hrt.2003.029470.

80. Tsai SH, Lu G, Xu X, Ren Y, Hein TW, Kuo L. Enhanced endothelin-1/Rho-kinase signalling and coronary microvascular dysfunction in hypertensive myocardial hypertrophy. Cardiovasc Res. 2017;113(11):1329–37. https://doi.org/10.1093/cvr/cvx103.

81. Ford TJ, Stanley B, Good R, Rocchiccioli P, McEntegart M, Watkins S, Eteiba H, Shaukat A, Lindsay M, Robertson K, Hood S, McGeoch R, McDade R, Yii E, Sidik N, McCartney P, Corcoran D, Collison D, Rush C, McConnachie A, Touyz RM, Oldroyd KG, Berry C. Stratified medical therapy using invasive coronary function testing in angina: The CorMicA Trial. J Am Coll Cardiol. 2018;72(23 Pt A):2841–55. https://doi.org/10.1016/j.jacc.2018.09.006.

82. Fukumoto Y, Ito A, Uwatoku T, Matoba T, Kishi T, Tanaka H, Takeshita A, Sunagawa K, Shimokawa H. Extracorporeal cardiac shock wave therapy ameliorates myocardial ischemia in patients with severe coronary artery disease. Corona Artery Dis. 2006;17(1):63–70. https://doi.org/10.1097/00019501-200602000-00011.

Printed in the United States
by Baker & Taylor Publisher Services